THE
PEDIATRIC
CARDIOLOGY
HANDBOOK

D0645635

THE PEDIATRIC CARDIOLOGY HANDBOOK

SECOND EDITION

MYUNG K. PARK, MD, FAAP, FACC

On leave of absence from:
Professor of Pediatrics
Head, Division of Cardiology
University of Texas Health Science Center
San Antonio, Texas

Currently:
Professor and Chairman
Department of Pediatrics
Arabian Gulf University College of Medicine
Manama, Bahrain

M Mosby

St. Louis Baltimore Boston Carlsbad Chicago Naples New York Philadelphia Portland
London Madrid Mexico City Singapore Sydney Tokyo Toronto Wiesbaden

Mosby

Dedicated to Publishing Excellence

A Times Mirror
Company

Vice President and Publisher: Anne S. Patterson
Editor: Laura DeYoung
Associate Developmental Editor: Jennifer Byington Geistler
Project Manager: Deborah L. Vogel
Production Editor: Karen L. Allman
Designer: Pati Pye
Manufacturing Manager: Theresa Fuchs

SECOND EDITION

Copyright © 1997 by Mosby–Year Book, Inc.

Previous edition copyrighted 1991.

Printed in the United States of America
Composition by Graphic World, Inc.
Printing/binding by Malloy Lithographing

Mosby–Year Book, Inc.
11830 Westline Industrial Drive
St. Louis, Missouri 63146

96 97 98 99 00 / 9 8 7 6 5 4 3 2 1

Library of Congress Cataloging-in-Publication Data

Park, Myung K. (Myung Kun), 1934-
    The pediatric cardiology handbook / Myung K. Park.
        p.   cm.
    Includes bibliographical references and index.
    ISBN 0-8151-9005-0
    1. Pediatric cardiology—Handbooks, manuals, etc.   I. Title.
    [DNLM: 1. Cardiovascular Diseases—in infancy & childhood—
handbooks.   WS 39 P236p 1997]
RJ421.P38   1997
618.92′12—dc20
DNLM/DLC
for Library of Congress   96-9210
                                                                            CIP

NOTICE

Every effort has been made to ensure that the drug dosage schedules herein are accurate and in accord with the standards accepted at the time of publication. However, as new research and experience broaden our knowledge, changes in treatment and drug therapy occur. Therefore the reader is advised to check the product information sheet included in the package of each drug (s)he plans to administer to be certain that changes have not been made in the recommended dose or in the contraindications. This is of particular importance in regard to new or infrequently used drugs.

Dedicated to my lovely wife, Issun, and our sons, Douglas, Christopher, and Warren.

PREFACE

Since the publication of the first edition of *The Pediatric Cardiology Handbook,* important advances have been made in the diagnosis and management of children with congenital and acquired heart diseases. Advances made in infant cardiac surgery, in particular, have been extraordinary for correction and palliation of many defects, including the most complex lesions. These advances make it necessary to update and expand the handbook. Despite the major updating and expansion, the book maintains the original goal of providing pediatricians, family practitioners, housestaff, and medical students with a succinct practical information source.

Although updates and revisions have been made throughout the book, the most expansion is made in the section on electrocardiography in Chapter I, which is the section most often referred to by the readers. Additionally, a number of new figures have been added to facilitate in-depth understanding for the readers. The sections on individual congenital and acquired heart defects have been updated or rewritten with incorporation of the most recent diagnostic and therapeutic advances, especially the surgical advances in terms of timing, indications, type of surgeries, and the results. Discussions of cardiovascular infections, Kawasaki disease, cardiomyopathy, and neonates with cardiac problems have also been updated. The chapters on cardiac arrhythmias have been expanded beyond the format of this book to include a more detailed discussion on supraventricular tachycardia and premature ventricular contractions. Topics of chest pain, syncope, long QT syndrome, hyperlipidemia and management of surgical patients have been rewritten with appropriate expansion. In Chapter IX, drugs have been arranged in alphabetical order to facilitate quick reference and the number of drugs included has been increased.

The author is deeply indebted to Dae-Hwan Shin, PhD, a personal friend, for introducing me to the Microsoft Word program and helping me whenever I had problems with the computer. I would also like to thank Mrs. Diane Halim for typing and editing. Most of all, I thank my wife for her understanding my long period of preoccupation with the project, particularly during the period when we were busy preparing for a move abroad.

Myung K. Park, MD
San Antonio, Texas

FREQUENTLY USED ABBREVIATIONS

AR	Aortic regurgitation
AS	Aortic stenosis
ASD	Atrial septal defect
BBB	Bundle branch block
CAH	Combined atrial hypertrophy
CHD	Congenital heart disease or defect
CHF	Congestive heart failure
COA	Coarctation of the aorta
CPB	Cardiopulmonary bypass
CXR	Chest x-ray
DORV	Double-outlet right ventricle
Echo	Echocardiography
HLHS	Hypoplastic left heart syndrome
HOCM	Hypertrophic obstructive cardiomyopathy
IHSS	Idiopathic hypertrophic subaortic stenosis
IVC	Inferior vena cava
LA	Left atrium or left atrial
LAD	Left axis deviation
LAE	Left atrial enlargement
LAH	Left atrial hypertrophy
LBBB	Left bundle branch block
LICS	Left intercostal space
LLN	Lower limit of normal
LLSB	Lower left sternal border
LPA	Left pulmonary artery
LPL	Left precordial lead
L-R shunt	Left-to-right shunt
LRSB	Lower right sternal border
LSB	Left sternal border
LV	Left ventricle or left ventricular
LVH	Left ventricular hypertrophy

LVOT	Left ventricular outflow tract
MLSB	Mid-left sternal border
MPA	Main pulmonary artery
MR	Mitral regurgitation
MRSB	Mid-right sternal border
MS	Mitral stenosis
MVP	Mitral valve prolapse
PA	Pulmonary artery or posteroanterior
PAC	Premature atrial contraction
PAPVR	Partial anomalous pulmonary venous return
PAT	Paroxysmal atrial tachycardia
PBF	Pulmonary blood flow
PDA	Patent ductus arteriosus
PFO	Patent foramen ovale
PR	Pulmonary regurgitation
PS	Pulmonary stenosis
PV	Pulmonary vein or pulmonary venous
PVC	Premature ventricular contraction
PVM	Pulmonary vascular marking
PVOD	Pulmonary vascular obstructive disease
PVR	Pulmonary vascular resistance
RA	Right atrium or right atrial
RAD	Right axis deviation
RAE	Right atrial enlargement
RAH	Right atrial hypertrophy
RBBB	Right bundle branch block
RICS	Right intercostal space
RPA	Right pulmonary artery
RPL	Right precordial lead
R-L shunt	Right-to-left shunt
RV	Right ventricle or right ventricular
RVE	Right ventricular enlargement
RVH	Right ventricular hypertrophy
RVOT	Right ventricular outflow tract
S1	First heart sound
S2	Second heart sound
S3	Third heart sound
S4	Fourth heart sound
SBE	Subacute bacterial endocarditis
SEM	Systolic ejection murmur

S-P shunt	Systemic-to-pulmonary shunt
SVC	Superior vena cava
SVR	Systemic vascular resistance
SVT	Supraventricular tachycardia
TAPVR	Total anomalous pulmonary venous return
TGA	Transposition of the great arteries
TOF	Tetralogy of Fallot
TR	Tricuspid regurgitation
TS	Tricuspid stenosis
ULN	Upper limit of normal
ULSB	Upper left sternal border
URSB	Upper right sternal border
VSD	Ventricular septal defect
VT	Ventricular tachycardia
WPW	Wolff-Parkinson-White (syndrome)

CONTENTS

CHAPTER IV. ACQUIRED HEART DISEASE, 159

CHAPTER V. ARRHYTHMIAS AND ATRIOVENTRICULAR CONDUCTION DISTURBANCES, 196

CHAPTER VIII. MANAGEMENT OF CARDIAC SURGICAL PATIENTS, 288

CHAPTER IX. CARDIOVASCULAR DRUG DOSAGE, 307

APPENDIX, 338

ROUTINE CARDIAC EVALUATION IN CHILDREN

I

Initial evaluation of children with possible cardiac problems includes (1) history taking, (2) physical examination, (3) electrocardiographic (ECG) evaluation, and (4) CXR. The weight of information gained from these techniques varies with the type and severity of the disease.

I. HISTORY TAKING

Important cardiovascular histories of infants and children include prenatal, perinatal, postnatal, past, and family histories.

A. Gestational and Perinatal History

1. Maternal infection: rubella (in which PDA and PA stenosis are common cardiac malformations). Other viral infections early in pregnancy may be teratogenic. Vital infections in late pregnancy may cause myocarditis.
2. Maternal medications: Amphetamines, anticonvulsants, progesterone, and estrogen are highly suspected teratogens. Excessive maternal alcohol intake may cause fetal alcohol syndrome (in which VSD, PDA, ASD, and TOF are common).
3. Maternal illnesses: maternal diabetes increases the prevalence of CHD (TGA, VSD, and PDA) and cardiomyopathy. Both maternal lupus erythematosus and collagen diseases are associated with congenital heart block in the offspring. History of maternal CHD may

increase the prevalence of CHD in the offspring to more than 10%, compared with 1% in the general population (See Appendix, Table A-1).

B. Postnatal and Present History

1. Poor weight gain and delayed development (may be caused by CHF, severe cyanosis, or general dysmorphic conditions).
2. Cyanosis, squatting, and cyanotic spells (suggest TOF and other cyanotic CHD).
3. Tachycardia, tachypnea, and puffy eyelids (signs of CHF).
4. Frequent lower respiratory tract infections (may be associated with large L-R shunt lesions).
5. Poor exercise tolerance (may be a sign of significant heart defects).
6. Heart murmur (age when first heard, any association with fever).
7. Chest pain (related to activity? duration, nature, and radiation. Cardiac origin of chest pain is usually associated with activity and/or history of known CHD) (see Chapter 7).
8. Palpitation (commonly caused by paroxysms of tachycardia or single premature beats).
9. Joint pain (joints involved, duration, migratory or stationary, recent sore throat, rashes, family history of rheumatic fever).
10. Neurologic symptoms: stroke from embolization or thrombosis from infective endocarditis or polycythemia; headache from polycythemia or hypertension (±); choreic movement from rheumatic fever. Fainting or syncope may be due to arrhythmias, long QT syndrome, or MVP (among other noncardiac conditions) (see Chapter 7).
11. Medications, cardiac and noncardiac (name, dosage, timing, duration).
12. Diseases of other systems with associated cardiovascular abnormalities (Tables 1-1 to 1-3).

TABLE 1-1.

Selected Syndromes and Diseases Associated
with Cardiovascular Abnormalities

Syndromes and Diseases	Incidence and Types of Cardiovascular Anomalies
Apert syndrome	Occasional; VSD, TOF
Carpenter syndrome	Occasional; PDA, VSD, PS, TGA
CHARGE association	Common (65%); conotruncal aomalies (TOF, truncus arteriosus), aortic arch anomalies (vascular ring, interrupted aortic arch)
Cockayne syndrome	Occasional; accelerated atherosclerosis
de Lange syndrome	Occasional (30%); VSD
Crouzon disease (craniofacial dysostosis)	Occasional; PDA, COA
DiGeorge syndrome (fourth branchial arch)	Common; interrupted aortic arch, truncus arteriosus, VSD, PDA, TOF
Ehlers-Danlos syndrome	Common; aneurysm of aorta and carotids
Ellis-van Creveld syndrome (chondro-ectodermal dysplasia)	Common (50%); single atrium
Fetal alcohol syndrome	Common (25%-30%); VSD, PDA, ASD, TOF
Friedreich's ataxia	Common; cardiomyopathy
Glycogen storage disease II (Pompe disease)	Very common; cardiomyopathy
Holt-Oram syndrome (cardiac limb)	Common; ASD, VSD
Homocystinuria syndrome	Common; medial degeneration of aorta and carotids, arterial or venous thrombus
HOCM	Hypertrophic obstructive subaortic stenosis
Kartagener syndrome	Dextrocardia
Laurence-Moon-Biedl syndrome	Occasional; VSD, other CHDs
Leopard syndrome	Very common; PS, long PR interval, cardiomyopathy
Long QT syndrome Jervell and Lange-Nielsen Romano-Ward	Very common; long QT interval, ventricular tachyarrhythmias

Continued.

TABLE 1-1.

Selected Syndromes and Diseases Associated
with Cardiovascular Abnormalities—cont'd

Syndromes and Diseases	Incidence and Types of Cardiovascular Anomalies
Marfan syndrome	Common; aortic aneurysm, AR, and/or MR
Mitral valve prolapse	Common; MR, arrhythmias
Mucopolysaccharidosis Hurler (type I) Hunter (type II) Morquio (type III)	Common; AR and/or MR, coronary artery disease
Muscular dystrophy (Duchenne type)	Common; cardiomyopathy
Neurofibromatosis (von Recklinghausen disease)	Occasional; PS, COA, pheochromocytoma
Noonan syndrome	Common; PS (dystrophic pulmonary valve), LVH or anterior septal hypertrophy
Osler-Weber-Rendu syndrome	Occasional; pulmonary AV fistula
Osteogenesis imperfecta	Occasional; aortic dilation, AR, MVP
Pierre Robin syndrome	Occasional (29%); VSD, PDA, less commonly ASD, COA, TOF
Progeria (Hutchinson-Gilford syndrome)	Common; accelerated atherosclerosis
Smith-Lemli-Opitz syndrome	Occasional; VSD, PDA, others
Thrombocytopenia and absent radius (TAR) syndrome	Occasional (33%); ASD, TOF, dextrocardia
Treacher Collins syndrome	Occasional; VSD, PDA, ASD
Tuberous sclerosis	Common; rhabdomyoma
VATER association	Common (>50%); VSD, other defects
von Hippel Lindau syndrome	Common; hemangiomas, pheochromocytoma with hypertension
Williams syndrome	Common; supravalvular AS, PA stenosis
Zellweger syndrome	Common; PDA, VSD, ASD

AV, atriovenous; PFC, persistent fetal circulation; PPHN, persistent pulmonary hypertension of newborn. Other abbreviations are listed on pp. ix–xi.

TABLE 1-2.

Congenital Heart Defects in Selected Chromosomal Aberrations

Condition	Prevalence	Common Defects in Decreasing Order of Frequency
5p–(cri du chat syndrome)	25%	VSD, PDA, ASD
Trisomy 13	90	VSD, PDA, dextrocardia
Trisomy 18	99	VSD, PDA, PS
Trisomy 21 (Down syndrome)	50	ECD, VSD
Turner syndrome (XO)	35	COA, AS, ASD
Klinefelter variant (XXXXY)	15	PDA, ASD

ECD, endocardial cushion defect. Other abbreviations are listed on pp. ix–xi.

C. Family History

1. Certain hereditary diseases may be associated with varying frequency of cardiac anomalies (Table 1-1).
2. CHD in the family. The incidence of CHD in the general population is about 1% (8 to 12 per 1000 live births). When one child is affected, the risk of recurrence in siblings is 3%. However, the risk of recurrence is related to the incidence of particular defects. Lesions with high prevalence (e.g., VSD) tend to have a high risk of recurrence, and those with low prevalence (e.g., tricuspid atresia, persistent truncus arteriosus) have a low risk of recurrence (see Appendix, Table A-2). The probability of recurrence is substantially higher when the mother rather than the father is the affected parent. Tables A-1 and A-2 can be used for counseling.
3. Rheumatic fever often occurs in more than one member of the family.

TABLE 1-3.

Incidence of Associated CHD in Patients with Other System Malformations

Organ System and Malformation	Incidence	Specific Cardiac Defect
Central Nervous System		
Hydrocephalus	6%	VSD, ECD, TOF
Dandy-Walker syndrome	3	VSD
Agenesis of corpus callosum	15	No specific defect
Meckel-Gruber syndrome	14	No specific defect
Thoracic Cavity		
TE fistula, esophageal atresia	21	VSD, ASD, TOF
Diaphragmatic hernia	11	No specific defect
Gastrointestinal System		
Duodenal atresia	17	No specific defect
Jejunal atresia	5	No specific defect
Anorectal anomalies	22	No specific defect
Imperforate anus	12	TOF, VSD
Ventral Wall		
Omphalocele	21	No specific defect
Gastroschisis	3	No specific defect
Genitourinary System		
Renal agenesis		
Bilateral	43	No specific defect
Unilateral	17	No specific defect
Horseshoe kidney	39	No specific defect
Renal dysplasia	5	No specific defect

ECD = endocardial cushion defect; TE, tracheoesophageal.
Adapted from Copel et al: Am J Obstet Gynecol 154:1121-1132, 1986.

II. PHYSICAL EXAMINATION

A. Inspection

1. General appearance: happy or cranky, nutritional state, respiratory status (tachypnea, dyspnea,

retraction may be signs of serious CHD), pallor (vaso-constriction from CHF, circulatory shock, or severe anemia), and sweat on the forehead (CHF).

2. Known syndromes and chromosomal abnormalities are listed in Tables 1-1 and 1-2.
3. Malformations of other systems may be associated with CHD (Table 1-3).
4. Cyanosis and clubbing. Cyanosis usually signals a serious CHD. A long-standing arterial desaturation (usually more than 6 months), even of a subclinical degree, results in clubbing of the fingernails and toenails.

B. Palpation

1. Precordium
   a. A hyperactive precordium is characteristic of heart diseases with high volume overload, such as L-R shunt lesions and severe valvular regurgitation.
   b. A thrill is often of real diagnostic value. The location of the thrill suggests certain cardiac anomalies: ULSB: PS, PA stenosis, and rarely PDA; URSB: AS; LLSB: VSD; suprasternal notch: AS, occasionally PS, PDA or COA; carotid arteries: AS, COA.
2. Peripheral pulses
   a. Check the peripheral pulse for the rate, irregularities (arrhythmias), and volume (bounding, full, or thready).
   b. Strong arm pulses and weak leg pulses suggest COA.
   c. The right brachial artery pulse stronger than the left brachial artery pulse may suggest COA or supravalvular AS.
   d. Bounding pulses are found in aortic runoff lesions (e.g., PDA, AR, large systemic AV fistula, rarely persistent truncus arteriosus).
   e. Weak, thready pulses are found in CHF and in circulatory shock.
   f. Pulsus paradoxus may be seen in patients with cardiac tamponade or constrictive pericarditis and in those on a respirator with a high pressure setting.

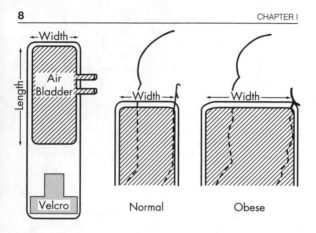

FIG. 1-1.
A method of selecting an appropriate-sized blood pressure cuff.
(From Park MK: *Pediatric cardiology for practitioners,* ed 3. St. Louis,
Mosby, 1995.)

C. Blood Pressure

The use of a correct-sized blood pressure (BP) cuff is
important. A narrow cuff will overestimate the true BP, and
a wide one will underestimate it. The width of the inflatable
part of the cuff (bladder) should be 40% to 50% of the
circumference (or 125% to 155% of the diameter) of the
arm or leg on which BP is to be determined (Fig 1-1), as
recommended by the American Heart Association (AHA).
Cuff selection based solely on the length of the arm (e.g.,
¾ of the length of the upper arm as recommended by the
National Institutes of Health [NIH] Task Force in 1987) is
scientifically unsound. The cuff should completely or
nearly completely encircle the limb.

For the auscultatory method phase I of the Korotkoff
sounds is taken as systolic pressure. The point of muffling
(phase IV) is taken as diastolic pressure in children 12 years
and younger and that of disappearance (phase V) in

TABLE 1-4.

Suggested Normative Blood Pressure Levels (mm Hg) by Auscultatory Method (systolic/diastolic K5)

Age (years)	Mean BP levels	90th percentile	95th percentile
6-7	104/55	114/73	117/78
8-9	106/58	118/76	120/82
10-11	108/60	120/77	124/82
12-13	112/62	124/78	128/83
14-15 boys	116/66	132/80	138/86
girls	112/68	126/80	130/83
16-18 boys	121/70	136/82	140/86
girls	110/68	125/81	127/84

BP values are adapted from Goldring et al: J Pediatrics 91:884-889, 1977; and Prineas et al: Hypertension 2 (suppl 1): 18-24, 1980. The BP cuff was selected to be 40% to 50% of the circumference of the upper arm. Values for ages 10 to 13 years have been extrapolated from these two studies using age-related increments from other studies.

children 13 years and older, but when they are more than 6 mm Hg apart, both values should be noted (such as 110/75/50 mm Hg). Although there is no single reliable set of normative BP values, a working guide of normal BP values is needed until more reliable data become available (Table 1-4).

The accuracy of indirect BP measurement by an oscillometric method (Dinamap) has been demonstrated. The cuff width 40% to 50% of the circumference (or 125% to 155% of the diameter) of the arm is also appropriate for the Dinamap method. Normal BP levels by the Dinamap method for newborns and children up to age 5 are presented in Table 1-5.

D. Auscultation

Systematic attention should be given to heart rate and regularity; intensity and quality of the heart sounds, especially the second heart sound; systolic and diastolic sounds (ejection click, midsystolic click, opening snap); and heart murmurs.

TABLE 1-5.

Normative Blood Pressure Levels (systolic/diastolic [mean]) (mm Hg) by Dinamap Monitor in Children up to Age 5

Age	Mean BP Levels	90th Percentile	95th Percentile
1-3 days	64/41 (50)	75/49 (59)	78/52 (62)
1 mo-2 yr	95/58 (72)	106/68 (83)	110/71 (86)
2-5 yr	101/57 (74)	112/66 (82)	115/68 (85)

Adapted from Park MK, Menard SM: Am J Dis Child 143:860-864, 1989.

1. Heart sounds
   a. The first heart sound (S1) is associated with closure of the mitral and tricupid valves and is best heard at the apex or LLSB. Splitting of the S1 is uncommon in normal children. Wide splitting of the S1 may be found in RBBB or Ebstein anomaly.
   b. The second heart sound (S2), which is produced by the closure of the aortic and pulmonary valves, is evaluated in the ULSB or the pulmonary area in terms of the degree of splitting and the relative intensity of the P2 (the pulmonary closure sound) in relation to the intensity of the A2 (the aortic closure sound). Although best heard with a diaphragm, both components are readily audible with the bell as well.
      1) The degree of splitting of the S2 normally varies with respiration, increasing with inspiration and decreasing or becoming single with expiration (Fig 1-2).
      2) Abnormal S2 may take the form of wide splitting, narrow splitting, single S2, abnormal intensity of the P2, or, rarely paradoxic splitting of the S2 (Table 1-6)
   c. The third heart sound (S3) is best heard at the apex or LLSB (Fig 1-3). It is commonly heard in normal children, young adults, and in patients with

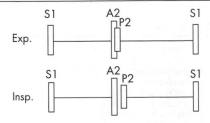

FIG. 1-2.
Relative intensity of the A2 and P2 and the respiratory variation in the degree of splitting of the S2 at the ULSB (pulmonary area). (From Park MK: *Pediatric cardiology for practitioners*, ed 3 St. Louis, Mosby, 1995.)

dilated ventricles and decreased compliance of the ventricles (e.g., large shunt VSD, CHF).
d. The fourth heart sound (S4) at the apex, which is always pathologic (Fig 1-3), is seen in conditions with decreased ventricular compliance or CHF.
e. Gallop rhythm generally implies pathology and results from the combination of a loud S3 or S4 and tachycardia. It is common in CHF.
2. Systolic and diastolic sounds
a. An ejection click sounds like splitting of the S1 but is best audible at the base rather than at the LLSB (Fig 1-3). The ejection click is associated with stenosis of the semilunar valves (e.g., PS at 2 to 3 LICS, AS at 2RICS or apex) and large great arteries (e.g., systemic hypertension; pulmonary hypertension; idiopathic dilation of the PA; TOF, in which the aorta is dilated; and persistent truncus arteriosus).
b. A midsystolic click with or without a late systolic murmur is heard near the apex in MVP (Fig 1-3).
c. Diastolic opening snap is audible at the apex or LLSB in mitral stenosis (Fig 1-3).

TABLE 1-6.

Summary of Abnormal S2

Abnormal splitting
1. Widely split and fixed S2
    a. Volume overload (ASD, PAPVR)
    b. Pressure overload (PS)
    c. Electrical delay (RBBB)
    d. Early aortic closure (MR)
    e. Occasional normal child
2. Narrowly split S2
    a. Pulmonary hypertension
    b. AS
    c. Occasional normal child
3. Single S2
    a. Pulmonary hypertension
    b. One semilunar valve (pulmonary atresia, aortic atresia, persistent truncus arteriosus)
    c. P2 not audible (TGA, TOF, severe PS)
    d. Severe AS
    e. Occasional normal child
4. Paradoxically split S2
    a. Severe AS
    b. LBBB, WPW syndrome (type B)
Abnormal intensity of P2
1. Increased P2 (pulmonary hypertension)
2. Decreased P2 (severe PS, TOF, tricuspid stenosis)

---

3. Heart murmur

Each heart murmur must be analyzed in terms of intensity, timing (systolic or diastolic), location, transmission, and quality (e.g., musical, vibratory, blowing).

1) Intensity of the murmur is customarily graded from 1 to 6.

Grade 1, barely audible.

Grade 2, soft but easily audible.

Grade 3, moderately loud but not accompanied by a thrill.

Grade 4, louder and associated with a thrill.

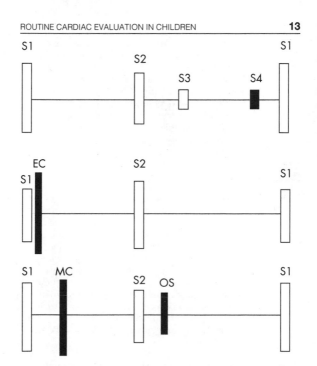

FIG. 1-3.
Relative position of the heart sounds, ejection click *(EC),* midsystolic click *(MC),* and diastolic opening snap *(OS).* Filled bars show abnormal sounds. (From Park MK: *Pediatric cardiology for practitioners,* ed 3 Mosby, St. Louis, 1995).

> Grade 5, audible with the stethoscope barely on the chest.
> Grade 6, audible with the stethoscope off the chest.

2) Classification of heart murmurs
   According to the timing of the heart murmur

in relation to S1 and S2, the heart murmur
is classified as systolic, diastolic, or continuous.

a. Systolic murmurs

  1) A systolic murmur occurs between S1 and S2
and is classified as one of two types, ejection
or regurgitant, depending on the timing of the
onset of the heart murmur in relation to the S1.

    a) Ejection systolic murmur (also called
stenotic, diamond-shaped,
crescendo-decrescendo murmur) has an
interval between S1 and the onset of the
murmur and is crescendo-decrescendo. The
murmur may be short or long (Fig 1-4, *A*).
These murmurs are caused by flow of blood
through stenotic or deformed semilunar
valves or increased flow through normal
semilunar valves and are therefore found
at the base or over the midprecordium.

    b) Regurgitant systolic murmur begins with the
S1 (no gap between the S1 and the onset of
the murmur) and usually lasts throughout
systole (pansystolic or holosystolic) but may
be decrescendo ending in middle or early
systole (Fig 1-4, *B*). These murmurs are associated with only three conditions: VSD, MR,
and TR.

  2) Location
In addition to the type of murmur (ejection vs.
regurgitant) the location of maximal intensity is
of great importance in determining the origin
(Tables 1-7 through 1-10, Fig 1-5).

  3) Transmission
A systolic ejection murmur at the base that
transmits well to the neck is likely to be aortic,
and one that transmits well to the sides of the
chest and the back is likely to arise in the
pulmonary valve or pulmonary artery.

  4) Quality
The quality of a murmur may be helpful in the
diagnosis of heart disease. Systolic murmurs

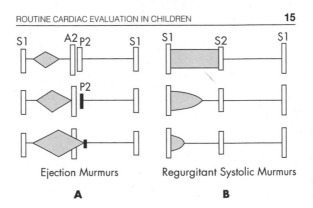

Ejection Murmurs   Regurgitant Systolic Murmurs

A   **B**

FIG. 1-4.
Ejection and regurgitant systolic murmurs. **A,** Ejection systolic murmurs audible in stenosis of the pulmonary valve. With mild stenosis the apex of the diamond is in the early part of systole *(top)*. With increasing severity of obstruction to flow the murmur becomes longer and its apex moves toward S2 *(middle)*. In severe PS the murmur may last beyond A2 *(bottom)*. **B,** Regurgitant systolic murmur starts with S1. Most regurgitant systolic murmur in children is due to VSD and is holosystolic, extending all the way to S2 *(top)*. In some children, especially those with small VSD and some newborns with VSD, the regurgitant systolic murmur ends in middle or early systole (not holosystolic) *(middle, bottom)*.

of MR or VSD have a uniform, high-pitched quality often described as blowing. Ejection systolic murmurs of AS or PS have a rough, grating quality. A common innocent murmur in children (Still murmur) has a characteristic vibratory or humming quality.

5) Differential diagnosis by location
Fig. 1-5 illustrates systolic murmurs that are audible at the various locations. Tables 1-7 through 1-10 summarize other important clinical findings (e.g., physical examination, CXR,

TABLE 1-7.

Differential Diagnosis of Systolic Murmurs at the ULSB (Pulmonary Area)

Condition	Important Physical Findings	Chest X-ray Findings	ECG Findings
PS	SEM grade 2-5/6 *Thrill (±) S2 may be split widely when mild *Ejection click (±) at 2LICS Transmit to back	*Prominent MPA (poststenotic dilation) Normal PVM	Normal if mild, RAD *RVH RAH if severe
ASD	SEM grade 2-3/6 *Widely split and fixed S2	*Increased PVM *RAE and RVE	RAD RVH *RBBB (rsR')
Pulmonary flow murmur of newborn	SEM grade 1-2/6 No thrill *Good transmission to back and axillae	Normal	Normal
Pulmonary flow murmur of older children	SEM grade 2-3/6 No thrill Poor transmission	Normal Occasional pectus ex-cavatum or straight back Prominent hilar vessels (±)	Normal
Pulmonary artery stenosis	SEM grade 2-3/6 Occasional continuous murmur P2 may be loud *Transmits well to back and both lung fields		RVH or normal

	Physical findings	Chest x-ray	ECG
AS	SEM grade 2-5/6 *Also audible in 2RICS *Thrill (±) at 2RICS and SSN *Ejection click at apex, 3LICS, or 2RICS (±) Paradox split S2 if severe	Dilated aorta	Normal or LVH
TOF	*Long SEM, grade 2-4/6 Louder at MLSB Thrill (±) Loud, single S2 (=A2) Cyanosis, clubbing	*Decreased PVM *Normal heart size Boot-shaped heart Right aortic arch (25%)	RAD *RVH or CVH RAH (±)
COA	SEM grade 1-3/6 *Loudest at left interscapular area (back) *Weak or absent femorals Hypertension in arms Frequently associated with AS, bicuspid aortic valve, or MR	*Classic 3 sign on plain film or E sign on barium esophagogram Rib notching (±)	LVH in children RBBB or RVH in newborns
PDA	*Continuous murmur, grade 2-4/6, at left infraclavicular area Occasional crescendic systolic only Thrill (±) Bounding pulses	*Increased PVM *LAE, LVE	Normal, LVH, or CVH

Continued.

TABLE 1-7.

Differential Diagnosis of Systolic Murmurs at the ULSB (Pulmonary Area)—cont'd

Condition	Important Physical Findings	Chest X-ray Findings	ECG Findings
TAPVR	SEM grade 2-3/6 Widely split and fixed S2 (±) *Quadruple or quintuple rhythm Diastolic rumble at LLSB *Mild cyanosis and clubbing (±)	*Increased PVM RAE and RVE Prominent MPA Snowman sign	RAD RAH *RVH
PAPVR	Physical findings similar to those of ASD *S2 may not be fixed unless associated with ASD	*Increased PVM *RAE and RVE Scimitar sign (±)	Same as in ASD

*Finding is particularly characteristic of the condition.
CVH, combined ventricular hypertrophy; 2LICS, second left intercostal space; SSN, suprasternal notch. Other abbreviations are listed on pp ix-xi.

TABLE 1-8.

Differential Diagnosis of Systolic Murmurs at the URSB (Aortic Area)

Condition	Important Physical Findings	Chest X-ray Findings	ECG Findings
Aortic valve stenosis	SEM grade 2-5/6 at 2RICS; may be loudest at 3LICS *Thrill (±), URSB, SSN, and carotid arteries *Ejection click *Transmits well to neck S2 may be single *AR murmur usually present	Mild LVE (±) Prominent ascending aorta or aortic knob	Normal or LVH with or without strain
Subaortic stenosis	SEM grade 2-4/6 No ejection click	Usually normal	Normal or LVH
Supravalvular aortic stenosis	SEM grade 2-3/6 Thrill (±) No ejection click *Pulse and BP may be greater in R than L arm *Peculiar facies, mental retardation (±) Murmur may transmit well to back (PA stenosis)	Unremarkable	Normal, LVH or CVH

*Finding is particularly characteristic of the condition.
CVH, combined ventricular hypertrophy; 3LICS, third left intercostal space; 2RICS, second right intercostal space; SSN, suprasternal notch. Other abbreviations are listed on pp ix-xi.

TABLE 1-9.

Differential Diagnosis of Systolic Murmurs at the LLSB

Condition	Important Physical Findings	Chest X-ray Findings	ECG Findings
VSD	*Regurgitant systolic, grade 2-5/6 May not be holosystolic Well localized at LLSB *Thrill often present P2 may be loud	*Increased PVM *LAE and LVE (cardiomegaly)	Normal LVH or CVH
Complete ECD	Similar to findings of VSD *Diastolic rumble at LLSB *Gallop rhythm common in infants (CHF)	Similar to large VSD	*Superior QRS axis, LVH or CVH
Vibratory innocent murmur (Still syndrome)	SEM grade 2-3/6 *Musical or vibratory with midsystolic accentuation *Maximum between LLSB and apex	Normal	Normal
HOCM or IHSS	SEM grade 2-4/6 Medium pitch Maximum LLSB or apex Thrill (±) *Sharp upstroke of brachial pulses May have MR murmur	Normal or globular LVE	LVH Abnormally deep Q waves in V5 and V6

Tricuspid regurgitation (TR)	*Regurgitant systolic, grade 2-3/6 *Triple or quadruple rhythm (in Ebstein anomaly) Mild cyanosis (±) Hepatomegaly with pulsatile liver and neck vein distention when severe	Normal PVM RAE if severe	RBBB, RAH, and first-degree AV block in Ebstein anomaly
Tetralogy of Fallot (TOF)	(See Table 1-7) Murmurs can be louder at ULSB		

*Finding is characteristic of the condition.
CVH, combined ventricular hypertrophy; ECD, endocardial cushion defect. Other abbreviations are listed on pp ix-xi.

TABLE 1-10.

Differential Diagnosis of Systolic Murmurs at the Apex

Condition	Important Physical Findings	Chest X-ray Findings	ECG Findings
MR	*Regurgitant systolic, may not be holosystolic, grade 2-3/6 Transmits to left axilla (less obvious in children) May be loudest in the midprecordium	LAE and LVE	LAH or LVH
MVP	*Midsystolic click with or without late systolic murmur *High incidence (85%) of thoracic skeletal anomalies (e.g., pectus excavatum, straight back)	Normal	Inverted T in aVF
AS	Murmur and ejection click may be best heard at apex rather than at 2RICS	(See Table 1-7)	
HOCM or IHSS	Murmur of IHSS may be maximal at apex (may represent MR) (See Table 1-9)		
Vibratory innocent murmur	This innocent murmur may be loudest at apex (See Table 1-9)		

*Finding is characteristic of the condition.
Abbreviations are listed on pp ix-xi.

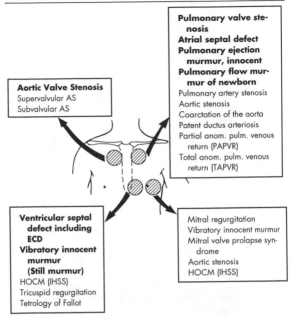

Aortic Valve Stenosis
Supervalvular AS
Subvalvular AS

Pulmonary valve stenosis
Atrial septal defect
Pulmonary ejection murmur, innocent
Pulmonary flow murmur of newborn
Pulmonary artery stenosis
Aortic stenosis
Coarctation of the aorta
Patent ductus arteriosis
Partial anom. pulm. venous return (PAPVR)
Total anom. pulm. venous return (TAPVR)

Ventricular septal defect including ECD
Vibratory innocent murmur (Still murmur)
HOCM (IHSS)
Tricuspid regurgitation
Tetrology of Fallot

Mitral regurgitation
Vibratory innocent murmur
Mitral valve prolapse syndrome
Aortic stenosis
HOCM (IHSS)

FIG. 1-5.
Systolic murmurs audible at various locations. More common conditions are shown in **boldface** type (see also Tables 1-7 through 1-10). (From Park MK: *Pediatric cardiology for practitioners,* ed 3, St. Louis, Mosby, 1995.)

and ECG) that may aid diagnosis according to the location of a systolic murmur.

b. Diastolic murmurs
Diastolic murmurs occur between S2 and S1. They have three types: early diastolic, middiastolic, and late diastolic.

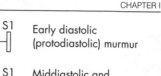

FIG. 1-6.
Diastolic murmurs and the continuous murmur. (From Park MK: *Pediatric cardiology for practitioners,* ed 3, St. Louis, Mosby, 1995.)

1) Early diastolic (protodiastolic) decrescendo murmurs are caused by AR or PR (Fig 1-6). AR murmurs are high pitched, are best heard with the diaphragm of the stethoscope at the 3LICS, and radiate to the apex. PR murmurs are usually medium pitched but may be high if pulmonary hypertension is present. Best heard at the 2LICS, they radiate along the left sternal border.

2) Middiastolic murmurs, which are always low pitched, start with a loud S3 (Fig 1-6). Best heard with the bell of the stethoscope, these murmurs are caused by anatomic or relative stenosis of the mitral or tricuspid valves. MS murmurs are best heard at the apex (apical rumble) and TS murmurs are heard along the LLSB.

3) Presystolic, or late diastolic, murmurs are low pitched and occur late in diastole or just before the onset of systole (Fig 1-6). They are found with anatomic stenosis of the mitral or tricuspid valve.

c. Continuous murmurs

Continuous murmurs begin in systole and continue without interruption through the S2 into all or part of diastole (Fig 1-6). Continuous murmurs are caused by the following:

1) Aortopulmonary or arteriovenous connection (e.g., PDA, atriovenous [AV] fistula, after S-P shunt surgery, or rarely, persistent truncus arteriosus).
2) Disturbances of flow patterns in veins (venous hum).
3) Disturbances of flow patterns in arteries (COA, peripheral PA stenosis). A combined systolic and diastolic murmur, such as from AS and AR or PS and PR, is called a to-and-fro murmur to distinguish it from a machinery-like continuous murmur.

d. Innocent murmurs

Over 80% of children have innocent murmurs of one type or the other sometime during childhood, most commonly beginning about 3 or 4 years of age. All innocent heart murmurs are accentuated or brought out in high-output states, most importantly with fever, and are associated with normal ECG and x-ray findings. Clinical characteristics of these murmurs are summarized in Table 1-11.

When one or more of the following are present, the murmur is likely to be pathologic and require cardiac consultation: (1) symptoms, (2) cyanosis, (3) abnormal CXR (heart size and/or silhouette and pulmonary vascularity), (4) abnormal ECG, (5) a systolic murmur that is loud (grade 3/6 or with a thrill) and long in duration, (6) a diastolic murmur, (7) abnormal heart sounds, and (8) abnormally strong or weak pulses.

III. ELECTROCARDIOGRAPHY

One normal cardiac cycle is represented by successive waveforms on an ECG tracing: the P wave, QRS complex, and the T wave (Fig 1-7, A). These waves produce two important intervals, RP and QT, and two segments, PQ and ST.

TABLE 1-11.

Common Innocent Heart Murmurs

Type (Timing)	Description of Murmur	Age Group
Classic vibratory murmur (Still murmur) (systolic)	Maximal at MLSB or between LLSB and apex Grade 2-3/6 Low-frequency vibratory, twanging string, groaning, squeaking, or musical	3-6 yr Occasionally in infancy
Pulmonary ejection murmur (systolic)	Maximal at ULSB Early to midsystolic Grade 1-3/6 in intensity Blowing in quality	8-14 yr
Pulmonary flow murmur of newborn (systolic)	Maximal at ULSB Transmits well to left and right chest, axillae, and back Grade 1-2/6 in intensity	Premature and full-term newborns Usually disappears by 3-6 mo of age
Venous hum (continuous)	Maximal at right (or left) supraclavicular and infraclavicular areas Grade 1-3/6 in intensity Inaudible in supine position Intensity changes with rotation of head and compression of jugular vein	3-6 yr
Carotid bruit (systolic)	Right supraclavicular area and over carotids Grade 2-3/6 in intensity Occasional thrill over carotid	Any age

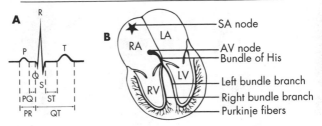

FIG. 1-7.
Definition of ECG configuration (**A**) and diagrammatic representation of the conduction system of the heart (**B**). (From Park MK, Guntheroth WG: *How to read pediatric ECGs,* ed 3, Mosby, St. Louis, 1992.)

In normal sinus rhythm the sinoatrial (SA) node is the pacemaker for the entire heart; the SA node impulse depolarizes the right and left atria by a contiguous spread, producing the P wave (Fig 1-7, A, B). When the atrial impulse arrives at the AV node, it passes through the node much more slowly than any other part of the heart, producing the PQ interval. Once the electrical impulse reaches the bundle of His, conduction becomes very fast and spreads simultaneously down the left and right bundle branches to the ventricular muscle through the Purkinje fibers, producing the QRS complex. The repolarization of the ventricle produces the T wave, but the repolarization of the atria is not usually visible on the ECG tracing.

A. Normal Pediatric Electrocardiograms

ECGs of normal infants and children are different from those of normal adults. The RV dominance in the ECG of newborns and infants is the result of the fetal circulation. The RV dominance is most marked in the newborn and is gradually replaced by the LV dominance of later childhood and adulthood. By age 3 to 4 years, pediatric ECGs resemble those of the adult. Figs 1-8 and 1-9 are ECGs from a newborn and an adult, respectively. The pediatric

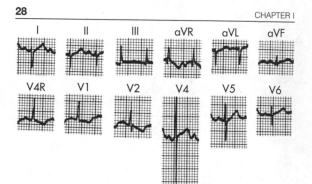

FIG. 1-8.
ECG of a normal newborn infant.

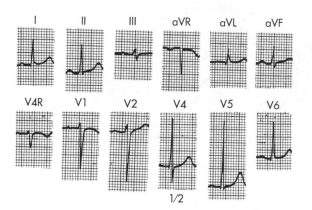

FIG. 1-9.
ECG of a normal young adult.

ECG has the following characteristics:

1. The heart rate is faster than in the adult.
2. All the durations and intervals (PR interval, QRS duration, QT interval) are shorter than in the adult. These intervals and durations increase with age.
3. The RV dominance of the newborn and infant is expressed in the ECG by the following:
   a. RAD.
   b. Large rightward forces (tall R waves in aVR and the right precordial leads [RPLs, i.e., V4R, V1, and V2] and deep S waves in lead I and the left precordial leads [LPLs, I.e., V5 and V6]).
   c. The R/S ratios in the RPLs are large and those in the LPLs are small. The R/S ratio is the ratio of the R amplitude and the S amplitude in a given lead.
   d. The T wave is inverted in V1 in infants and small children with the exception of the first 3 days when the T waves may be normally upright.

B. Vectorial Approach to the ECG

The ECG waves represent the direction and amplitude of the electromotive forces of the heart. The vectorial approach clarifies the meaning of the ECG waves and the concept of axes, such as the P axis, QRS axis, and T axis. The frontal view of the electrical activity (hexaxial reference system) is represented by the six limb leads (i.e., leads I, II, III, aVR, aVL and aVF), and the horizontal plane activity (horizontal reference system) is represented by the precordial leads (V1 through V6). When these two views are combined, a three-dimensional description of the electrical activity of the heart can be obtained (i.e., vector) in terms of the direction and the magnitude.

The *hexaxial reference system* shows the frontal view of the electrical activity as in the frontal plane of a vectorcardiography. This system, which uses the six limb leads, gives information about the left-right and superoinferior relationship (Fig 1-10, A). The positive pole of each lead is indicated by the lead labels. The positive deflection (i.e.,

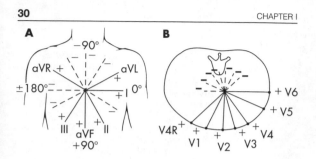

FIG. 1-10.
A, Hexaxial reference system. **B,** Horizontal reference system.
(Adapted from Park MK: Guntheroth WG: *How to read pediatric ECGs,* ed 3, St. Louis, Mosby, 1992.)

the R wave) is the force directed to the positive pole, and the negative deflection (i.e., the S wave) is the force directed toward the negative pole. Therefore the R wave in lead I represents the leftward force and the S wave in lead I the rightward force. The R wave in a VF is the inferior force, and the S wave in the same lead represents the superior force. The R wave in lead II is the left and inferior force, and the R wave in lead III is the right and inferior force. Upright P waves in lead I and aVF indicate that the P vector is directed left and inferiorly (as seen in sinus rhythm). It is necessary to memorize the hexaxial system. An easy way is shown in Fig 1-11 by a superimposition of a body with stretched arms and legs on the X and Y axes. The hands and feet are the positive poles of certain leads. The left and right hands are the positive poles of leads aVR and aVL, respectively. The left and right feet are the positive poles of leads II and III, respectively. The bipolar limb leads I, II, and III are clockwise in sequence for the positive poles.

While the hexaxial reference system gives information about the left-right and superior-inferior relationships, the *horizontal reference system* gives information about the anteroposterior and left-right relationship. The horizontal reference system uses precordial leads (e.g., V1, V2, V5,

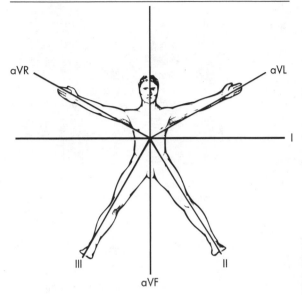

FIG. 1-11.
Easy way to memorize the hexaxial reference system.

V6) (Fig 1-10, B). The positive poles of the precordial leads are marked by the lead labels. The R wave in V2 represents the anterior force and the S wave in the same lead represents the posterior force. The R wave in V6 is the leftward force and the S wave in the same lead is the rightward force. The R wave in V1 is the right and anterior force and the S wave in this lead is the posterior and leftward force.

C. Routine Interpretation

The following sequence is one of many approaches that can be used in routine interpretation of an ECG.

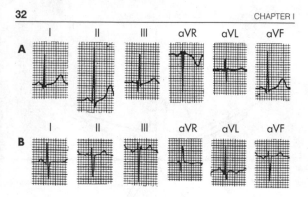

FIG. 1-12.
Sinus or nonsinus rhythm determined by the P axis. **A,** sinus rhythm
with the P axis between 0 and +90 degrees. **B,** a nonsinus rhythm
with the P axis in the 0 to –90 degrees quadrant. The presence of a
P wave in front of each QRS complex does not necessarily mean the
rhythm is sinus rhythm; the P axis should be in the normal quadrant,
as in **A.**

    a. Rhythm (sinus or nonsinus), considering the P
       axis.
    b. Heart rate (atrial and ventricular rates, if differ-
       ent).
    c. The QRS axis, the T axis, and the QRS-T angle.
    d. Intervals: PR, QRS, and QT.
    e. The P wave amplitude and duration.
    f. The QRS amplitude and R/S ratio; also note ab-
       normal Q waves.
    g. ST segment and T wave abnormalities.
1. Rhythm
  Sinus rhythm, the normal rhythm at any age,
  must meet the following two characteristics (Fig
  1-12, A):
  a. A P wave preceding each QRS complex with a
    regular PR interval. (The PR interval may be
    prolonged as in first-degree AV block.)
  b. The P axis between 0 and +90 degrees (with up-

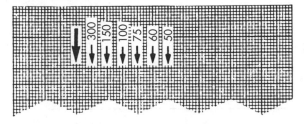

FIG. 1-13.
Quick method of estimating heart rate.

right P waves in leads I and aVF). This is important in discriminating sinus from nonsinus rhythm.
Some atrial (nonsinus) rhythm may have P waves
in front of each QRS complex but with an abnormal P axis (i.e., outside the 0 to +90 degree quadrant) (Fig 1-12, B). For the P axis to be between
0 and +90 degrees, P waves must be upright in
leads I and aVF; simple inspection of these two
leads suffices (Fig 1-10, A). A normal P axis (seen
in sinus rhythm) produces an upright P wave in
lead II and an inverted P wave in aVR.

2. Heart rate
  At the usual paper speed of 25 mm/sec, 1 mm = 0.04
  sec and 5 mm = 0.2 sec. The heart rate may be calculated by the following method.
  a. Measure the RR interval in seconds and divide 60
     by it.
  b. For quick estimation, inspect the RR interval in
     millimeters and use the following relationship: 5
     mm, 300/sec; 10 mm, 150/sec; 15 mm, 100/sec;
     20 mm, 75/sec; 25 mm, 60/sec (Fig 1-13).
  c. Use a convenient ECG ruler.
  The heart rate of children varies with age, status at the
time of ECG recording (awake, sleeping, crying, anxious),
and other physical factors such as fever. Normal resting
heart rates per minute according to age are shown in
Table 1-12.

TABLE 1-12.

Normal Ranges of Resting Heart Rate

Age	Beats/Min
Newborns	110-150
2 yr	85-125
4 yr	75-115
Over 6 yr	60-100

Tachycardia is a heart rate faster than the upper range of normal, and bradycardia is a heart rate slower than the low range of normal for that age.

3. The QRS axis, the T axis, and the QRS-T angle

   a. A convenient way of determining the QRS axis is by the use of the hexaxial reference system (Fig 1-10, A).

Successive Approximation Method

Step 1. Locate a quadrant using leads I and aVF (Fig 1-14).

Step 2. Find a lead with equiphasic QRS complex (in which the height of the R wave and the depth of the S wave are equal). The QRS axis is perpendicular to the lead with equiphasic QRS complex in the predetermined quadrant.

Example 1. Determine the QRS axis in Fig 1-15, A.

Step 1. The axis is in the left lower quadrant (0 to +90 degrees), since the R waves are upright in both leads I and aVF.

Step 2. The QRS complex is equiphasic in aVL. Therefore the QRS axis is +60 degrees, which is perpendicular to aVL (Fig 1-15, B).

Example 2. Determine the QRS axis in Fig 1-16, A.

Step 1. The QRS complexes are negative in lead I and negative in aVF, placing the axis in the right upper quadrant (−90 to −180 degrees) (Fig 1-14).

Step 2a. It is almost equiphasic in aVL but slightly more positive. Therefore the axis is close to −120 degrees.

Step 2b. Lead II has the deepest negative deflection. The negative limb of lead II is −120 degrees. The

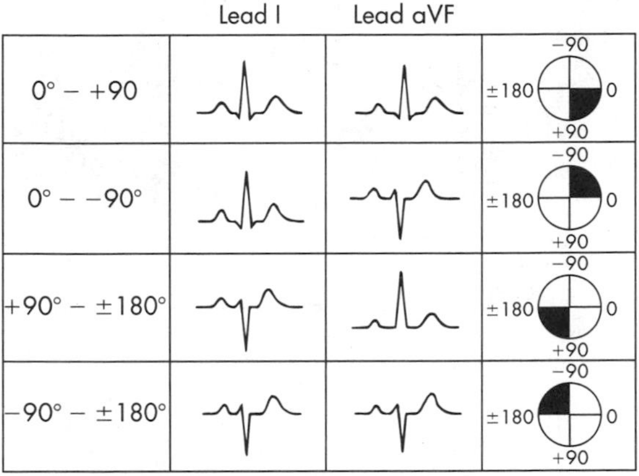

FIG. 1-14.
Locating quadrants of mean QRS axis from leads I and aVF. (From Park MK, Guntheroth WG: *How to read pediatric ECGs,* ed 3, St. Louis, Mosby, 1992.)

axis is *indeterminate,* that is, neither right nor left. The normal QRS axis varies with age (Table 1-13). The abnormal QRS axis has the following significance:

1) LAD with the QRS axis less than the lower limits of normal is seen in LVH, LBBB, and left anterior hemiblock (or superior QRS axis, characteristically seen with ECD and tricuspid atresia).

2) RAD, with the QRS axis greater than the upper limits of normal, is seen in RVH and RBBB.

3) Superior QRS axis is present when the S wave is greater than the R wave in aVF. It includes the left anterior hemiblock (in the range of −30 degrees to −90 degrees) and extreme RAD.

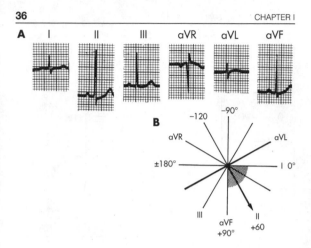

FIG. 1-15.
A, top, **B,** bottom right.

> b. The T axis can be determined by the methods used to determine the QRS axis.
>
> Example: Determine the T axis in Fig 1-16, A.
>
> In Fig 1-16, A, the positive T wave in lead I and the positive T wave in aVF place the T axis in the left lower quadrant (0 to +90 degrees). The T wave is nearly flat in aVL, and therefore the T axis is perpendicular to this lead, close to +60 degrees (or the positive pole of lead II, which shows the tallest T wave).
>
> The normal T axis is 0 to +90 degrees.
>
> The abnormal T axis (outside 0 to +90 degrees quadrant) is present when the T wave is inverted in lead I or aVF, usually resulting in a wide QRS-T angle. An abnormal QRS axis suggests conditions with myocardial dysfunction (myocarditis, myocardial ischemia), ventricular hypertrophy with strain, or RBBB.

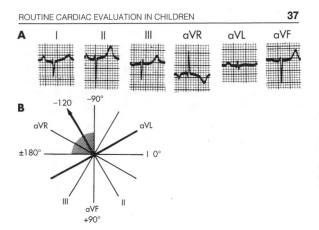

FIG. 1-16.
A, top, B, bottom left.

TABLE 1-13.

Mean and Range of Normal QRS Axes

1 wk–1 mo	+110 degrees (+30-+180)
1–3 mo	+70 degrees (+10-+125)
3 mo–3 yr	+60 degrees (+10-+110)
>3 yr	+60 degrees (+20-+120)
Adults	+50 degrees (−30-+105)

    c. The QRS-T angle is the angle formed by the QRS axis and the T axis. In Fig 1-16, the QRS-T angle is about 180 degrees. (The QRS axis is −120 degrees, and the T axis is about +60 degrees.)

        The normal QRS-T angle is less than 60 degrees except in the newborn period, when it may be more than 60 degrees.

The QRS-T angle of more than 60 degrees is unusual and that of more than 90 degrees is certainly abnormal. The abnormal QRS-T angle (above 90 degrees) is seen in severe ventricular hypertrophy with strain, ventricular conduction disturbances, and myocardial dysfunction of a metabolic or ischemic nature.

4. Intervals

a. The PR interval is measured from the onset of the P wave to the beginning of the QRS complex.

The normal PR interval varies with age and heart rate (Table 1-14). The older the person and the slower the heart rate, the longer is the PR interval.

A prolonged PR interval (first degree AV block) may be seen in conditions with myocardial dysfunction, viral or rheumatic, myocarditis, certain CHD (ECD, ASD, Ebstein anomaly), digitalis toxicity, hyperkalemia, and in an otherwise normal heart. A short PR interval is present in preexcitation (Wolff-Parkinson-White [WPW] syndrome, Lown-Ganong-Levine syndrome) and glycogen storage disease. Variable PR intervals are seen in wandering atrial pacemaker and Wenckebach (Mobitz type I) second-degree AV block.

b. Normal QRS duration varies with age (Table 1-15). A prolonged QRS is characteristic of ventricular conduction disturbances, which include bundle branch blocks (BBBs), preexcitation (WPW syndrome), intraventricular block, and ventricular arrhythmias (Fig 1-17). A slight prolongation of the QRS duration may be seen in ventricular hypertrophy.

c. The QT interval normally varies primarily with heart rate. The heart rate–corrected QT interval (QTc) can be calculated with Bazett's formula:

$$QT_c = QT/\sqrt{RR\ interval}$$

Normal QTc interval does not exceed 0.44 sec except in infants. A QTc up to 0.49 sec may be normal for the first 6 months of age.

TABLE 1-14.

PR Interval with Rate, Age (Upper Limits of Normal)

Rate	0-1 mo	1-6 mo	6 mo-1 yr	1-3 yr	3-8 yr	8-12 yr	12-16 yr	Adult
<60								0.17 (0.21)
60-80	0.10 (0.12)							0.16 (0.21)
80-100	0.10 (0.12)					0.16 (0.18)	0.16 (0.19)	0.15 (0.20)
100-120	0.10 (0.11)				0.15 (0.17)	0.15 (0.17)	0.15 (0.18)	0.15 (0.19)
120-140	0.09 (0.11)	0.11 (0.14)	0.11 (0.14)	(0.15)	0.14 (0.16)	0.15 (0.16)	0.15 (0.17)	0.15 (0.18)
140-160	0.10 (0.11)	0.10 (0.13)	0.11 (0.13)	0.12 (0.14)	0.13 (0.16)	0.14 (0.15)	0.15 (0.16)	(0.17)
160-180	0.10 (0.11)	0.10 (0.12)	0.10 (0.12)	0.11 (0.14)	0.13 (0.15)	0.14 (0.15)		
>180	0.09	0.09 (0.11)	0.10 (0.11)	0.10 (0.12)	0.12 (0.14)			

From Park MK, Guntheroth WG: How to Read Pediatric ECGs, ed 3. St. Louis, Mosby, 1992.

TABLE 1-15.

QRS Duration: Average (and Upper Limits) for Age

	0-1 mo	1-6 mo	6 mo-1 yr	1-3 yr	3-8 yr	8-12 yr	12-16 yr	Adult
Seconds	0.05 (0.07)	0.05 (0.07)	0.05 (0.07)	0.06 (0.07)	0.07 (0.08)	0.07 (0.09)	0.07 (0.10)	0.08 (0.10)

Modified from Guntheroth WG: Pediatric Electrocardiography. Philadelphia, WB Saunders Co, 1965.

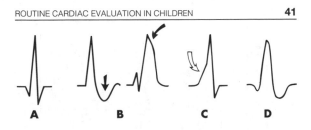

FIG. 1-17.
Schematic diagram of three types of ventricular conduction disturbances. **A,** normal QRS complex. **B,** QRS complexes in RBBB with terminal slurring *(black arrows).* **C,** preexcitation with delta wave *(initial slurring, open arrow).* **D,** intraventricular block in which the prolongation of the QRS complex is throughout the duration of the QRS complex. (From Park MK: *Pediatric cardiology for practitioners,* ed 3, St. Louis, Mosby, 1995.)

Long QT intervals may be seen in hypocalcemia, myocarditis, diffuse myocardial diseases, long QT syndrome (Jervell and Lange-Nielsen syndrome, Romano-Ward syndrome), head injury, and so on. A number of drugs can prolong the QTc interval, including antiarrhythmic drugs (class IA and III), antipsychotic phenothiazides (Mellaril, Thorazine), tricyclic antidepressants (imipramine, amitriptyline) antibiotics (e.g., ampicillin, erythromycin, trimethoprim-sulfamethoxazole, amantadine), antihistamine (Seldane), arsenics and organophosphates. A short QT interval is a sign of digitalis effect or of hypercalcemia.

5. P wave duration and amplitude
   Normally the P wave amplitude is less than 3 mm. The duration of the P waves is shorter than 0.09 sec in children and shorter than 0.07 sec in infants. Tall P waves indicate RAH. Long P wave durations are seen in LAH.
6. QRS amplitude, R/S ratio, and abnormal Q waves
   a. QRS amplitude varies with age (Table 1-16).

TABLE 1-16.

R and S Voltages According to Lead and Age: Mean (Upper Limits)*

Voltage	Lead	0-1 mo	1-6 mo	6 mo-1 yr	1-3 yr	3-8 yr	8-12 yr	12-16 yr	Young Adults
R wave	I	4 (8)	7 (13)	8 (16)	8 (16)	7 (15)	7 (15)	6 (13)	6 (13)
	II	6 (14)	13 (24)	13 (27)	13 (23)	13 (22)	14 (24)	14 (24)	9 (25)
	III	8 (16)	9 (20)	9 (20)	9 (20)	9 (20)	9 (24)	9 (24)	6 (22)
	aVR	3 (7)	3 (6)	3 (6)	2 (6)	2 (5)	2 (4)	2 (4)	1 (4)
	aVL	2 (7)	4 (8)	5 (10)	5 (10)	3 (10)	3 (10)	3 (12)	3 (9)
	aVF	7 (14)	10 (20)	10 (16)	8 (20)	10 (19)	10 (20)	11 (21)	5 (23)
	V4R	6 (12)	5 (10)	4 (8)	4 (8)	3 (8)	3 (7)	3 (7)	
	V1	15 (25)	11 (20)	10 (20)	9 (18)	7 (18)	6 (16)	5 (16)	3 (14)
	V2	21 (30)	21 (30)	19 (28)	16 (25)	13 (28)	10 (22)	9 (19)	6 (21)
	V5	12 (30)	17 (30)	18 (30)	19 (36)	21 (36)	22 (36)	18 (33)	12 (33)
	V6	6 (21)	10 (20)	13 (20)	13 (24)	14 (24)	14 (24)	14 (22)	10 (21)
S wave	I	5 (10)	4 (9)	4 (9)	3 (8)	2 (8)	2 (8)	2 (8)	1 (6)
	V4R	4 (9)	4 (12)	5 (12)	3 (12)	5 (14)	6 (20)	6 (20)	
	V1	10 (20)	7 (18)	8 (16)	13 (27)	14 (30)	16 (26)	15 (24)	10 (23)
	V2	20 (35)	16 (30)	17 (30)	21 (34)	23 (38)	23 (38)	23 (48)	14 (36)
	V5	9 (30)	9 (26)	8 (20)	6 (16)	5 (14)	5 (17)	5 (16)	1 (13)
	V6	4 (12)	2 (7)	2 (6)	2 (6)	1 (5)	1 (4)	1 (5)	

Modified from Park MK, Guntheroth WG: How to read pediatric ECGs, ed 3, St. Louis, Mosby, 1992.
Voltages measured in millimeters, when 1 mV = 10 mm paper.

1) Large QRS amplitudes are found in ventricular hypertrophy and ventricular conduction disturbances (e.g., BBBs, WPW syndrome).
2) Low QRS voltages are seen in pericarditis, myocarditis, hypothyroidism, and normal newborns.

b. In normal infants and small children, the R/S ratio is large in the RPLs and is small in the LPLs because of tall R waves in the RPLs and deep S waves in the LPLs (Table 1-17). Abnormal R/S ratios are seen in ventricular hypertrophy and ventricular conduction disturbances.

c. Normal Q waves are narrow (0.02 sec) and are usually less than 5 mm in LPLs and aVF. They may be as deep as 8 mm in lead III in children younger than 3 years old. Q waves are normally absent in RPLs.
1) Deep Q waves may be present in the LPLs in ventricular hypertrophy of the volume overload type.
2) Deep and wide Q waves are seen in myocardial infarction and myocardial fibrosis.
3) Q waves in V1 may be seen in severe RVH, ventricular inversion (L-TGA), single ventricle, and occasional newborns.
4) Absent Q waves in V6 may be seen in LBBB and ventricular inversion.

7. ST segment and T waves
a. The normal ST segment is isoelectric. However, in infants and children, elevation or depression of the ST segment up to 1 mm in the limb leads and up to 2 mm in the left precordial leads are not necessarily abnormal. J depression is a nonpathologic ST segment shift in which the junction between the QRS and the ST segment (i.e., J point) is depressed without sustained ST segment depression (Fig 1-18, A).

An abnormal shift of the ST segment assumes either a downward slope of the ST segment followed by a diphasic inverted T wave or a sustained horizontal segment 0.08 sec or longer (Fig 1-18, B, C). A pathologic ST segment shift is discussed

TABLE 1-17.
R/S Ratio According to Age: Mean, Lower, and Upper Limits of Normal

Lead		0-1 mo	1-6 mo	6 mo-1 yr	1-3 yr	3-8 yr	8-12 yr	12-16 yr	Adult
V1	LLN	0.5	0.3	0.3	0.5	0.1	0.15	0.1	0.0
	Mean	1.5	1.5	1.2	0.8	0.65	0.5	0.3	0.3
	ULN	19	S = 0	6	2	2	1	1	1
V2	LLN	0.3	0.3	0.3	0.3	0.05	0.1	0.1	0.1
	Mean	1	1.2	1	0.8	0.5	0.5	0.5	0.2
	ULN	3	4	4	1.5	1.5	1.2	1.2	2.5
V6	LLN	0.1	1.5	2	3	2.5	4	2.5	2.5
	Mean	2	4	6	20	20	20	10	9
	ULN	S = 0	S = 0	S = 0	S = 0	S = 0	S = 0	S = 0	S = 0

From Guntheroth WG: Pediatric electrocardiography. Philadelphia, WB Saunders Co, 1965. Used by permission.

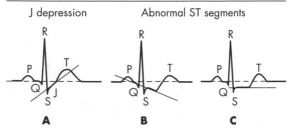

FIG. 1-18.
Nonpathologic (nonischemic) and pathologic (ischemic) ST and T changes. **A,** Characteristic nonischemic ST segment alteration called J depression; note that the ST slope is upward. **B, C,** ischemic or pathologic ST segment alterations. **B,** Downward slope of the ST segment. **C,** Horizontal segment is sustained.

later in this chapter. It occurs in pericarditis, myocardial ischemia or infarction, severe ventricular hypertrophy (with strain), and digitalis effect. Associated T wave changes are commonly present.

b. Tall peaked T waves may be seen in hyperkalemia, LVH (volume overload) and cerebrovascular accident (CVA). Flat or low T waves may occur in normal newborns or with such conditions as hypothyroidism, hypokalemia, digitalis, pericarditis, myocarditis, myocardial ischemia, hyperglycemia, or hypoglycemia.

D. Atrial Hypertrophy

Abnormalities in the P wave amplitude and/or duration characterize atrial hypertrophy.

1. RAH accompanies tall P waves (at least 3 mm).
2. LAH accompanies wide P wave duration (at least 0.1 sec in children and >0.08 sec in infants).
3. CAH accompanies a combination of tall and wide P wave.

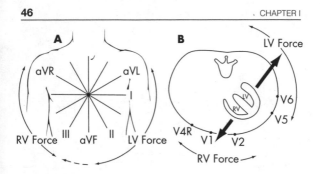

FIG. 1-19.
Left and right ventricular forces on the frontal projection. **A,** Hexaxial reference system. **B,** Horizontal plane.

E. Ventricular Hypertrophy

Ventricular hypertrophy produces abnormalities in one or more of the following: the QRS axis, the QRS voltages, the R/S ratio, the T axis, and miscellaneous changes.

1. The QRS axis is usually directed toward the hypertrophied ventricle (see Table 1-13 for normal QRS axis).
2. QRS voltages increase toward the hypertrophied ventricle (Table 1-16). In the frontal plane the LV mass lies to the left inferior to the cardiac center of gravity, and the RV lies to the right and inferior. Therefore, in LVH, the R wave amplitude increases in leads I, II, aVL, aVF, and sometimes III in the frontal plane (Fig 1-19, A). In RVH the R voltages increase in aVR and III, and the S voltages increase in lead I (Fig 1-19, A). An abnormally deep S wave in lead I is a reliable and reproducible sign of RVH, but abnormally deep S waves in V5 and V6 are sometimes due to imprecise placement of the chest lead electrodes. In the horizontal plane the RV occupies the right and anterior aspect and the LV the left and posterior aspect of the ventricular mass. Therefore, in RVH the R voltages in V4R, V1, and V2, as well as the S voltages in V5 and

V6, increase. In LVH, the R voltages in V5 and V6 and the S voltage in V1 and V2 increase. The R waves in V1 reflect a rightward and anterior force, and the increased R voltage in V1 is a reliable sign of RVH.

3. Changes in R/S ratio: An increase in the R/S ratio in the RPLs suggests RVH and a decrease in the ratio in these leads suggests LVH. An increase in the R/S ratio in the LPLs suggests LVH and a decrease in the ratio suggests RVH (Table 1-17).

4. Changes in the T axis: In severe ventricular hypertrophy with relative ischemia of the hypertrophied myocardium, the T axis changes. In the presence of criteria of ventricular hypertrophy, a wide QRS-T angle (90 degrees or greater) with the T axis outside the normal range indicates a strain pattern. When the T axis remains in the normal quadrant (0 to +90 degrees), a wide QRS-T angle indicates a possible strain pattern.

5. Miscellaneous nonspecific changes
   a. RVH: (1) A q wave in V1 (either qR or qRs) suggests RVH. (2) An upright T wave in V1 after 3 days of age is a sign of probable RVH.
   b. LVH: Deep Q waves (5 mm or greater) and/or tall T waves in V5 and V6 are signs of LVH of volume overload type (often seen with a large-shunt VSD).

   Criteria for Right Ventricular Hypertrophy: The more independent criteria for RVH that are satisfied, the more probable is RVH. An abnormal force both rightward and anterior is stronger evidence than one that is anterior only or rightward only. An example of RVH is shown in Fig 1-20.

   a. RAD for the patient's age (Table 1-13).
   b. Increased rightward and anterior QRS voltages in the presence of normal QRS duration.
      1) R in V1, V2, or aVR greater than the upper limits of normal for the patient's age (Table 1-16).
      2) S in I and V6 greater than the upper limits of normal for the patient's age (Table 1-16).
   c. Abnormal R/S ratio in favor of the RV in the absence of BBB (Table 1-17).

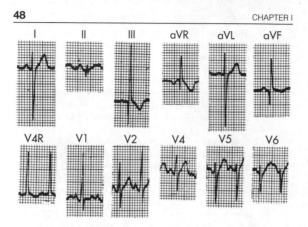

FIG. 1-20.
Tracing from a 10-month-old infant with severe TOF. The tracing shows RVH with strain. There is RAD (+150 degrees). The R waves in III (22 mm) and aVR (9 mm) and the S waves in I (19 mm) and V6 (8 mm) are abnormally large, indicating RVH. The R/S ratios in V1 and V2 are abnormally large, and the ratio in V6 is smaller than the LLN (Table 1-17), also indicating RVH. The S wave is inverted in aVF with the T axis of –10 degrees and a wide QRS-T angle (160 degrees).

     1) R/S ratio in V1 and V2 greater than the upper limits of normal for age.
     2) R/S ratio in V6 less than 1 after 1 month of age.
  d. Upright T in V1 in patients more than 3 days of age, provided that the T is upright in the LPLs (V5, V6). Upright T in V1 is not abnormal in patients 6 years or older.
  e. A q wave in V1 (qR or qRs patterns) suggests RVH.
  f. In the presence of RVH, a wide QRS-T angle with T axis outside the normal range (usually in the 0 to –90 degree quadrant) indicates a strain pattern.
    RVH in the Newborn: The diagnosis of RVH in the newborn is particularly difficult because of the

normal dominance of the RV during that period of life. The following clues, however, are helpful.

a. S waves in lead I, ≥12 mm.
b. R waves in aVR, ≥8 mm.
c. The following abnormalities in V1 also suggest RVH.
   1) Pure R wave (no S wave) in V1 greater than 10 mm.
   2) R in V1 ≥25 mm.
   3) A qR pattern in V1 (also seen in 10% of healthy newborn infants).
   4) Upright T waves in V1 in newborns more than 3 days of age with upright T in V6.
d. RAD greater than +180 degrees.

Criteria for Left Ventricular Hypertrophy: The more of the following independent criteria that are satisfied, the more probable is LVH. With obstructive lesions (e.g., AS), the abnormal force is more likely inferior. With a volume overload (e.g., VSD), the abnormal force is more likely to the left. An example of LVH is shown in Fig 1-21.

a. LAD for the patient's age (Table 1-13).
b. QRS voltages in favor of the LV in the presence of normal QRS duration.
   1) R in I, II, III, aVL, aVF, V5 or V6 greater than the upper limits of normal for age (Table 1-16).
   2) S in V1 or V2 greater than the upper limits of normal for age (Table 1-16).
c. Abnormal R/S ratio in favor of the LV: An R/S ratio in V1 and V2 less than the lower limits of normal for the patient's age (Table 1-17).
d. Q in V5 and V6, 5 mm or more, coupled with tall symmetric T waves in the same leads (volume overload type).
e. In the presence of LVH, a wide QRS-T angle with the T axis outside the normal range indicates a strain pattern. This is manifested by inverted T waves in lead I or aVF.

Criteria for Combined Ventricular Hypertrophy

a. Positive voltage criteria for RVH and LVH in the absence of BBB or WPW syndrome.

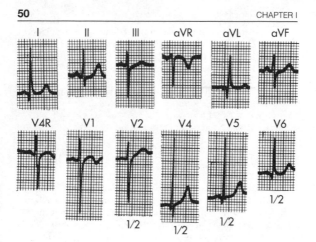

FIG. 1-21.
Tracing from a 4-year-old boy with moderate VSD. The tracing shows
LVH without strain pattern. The QRS axis is 0 degrees (LAD for age).
The R waves in I (17 mm), aVL (12 mm), V5 (44 mm), and V6 (27 mm)
are beyond the upper limits of normal, indicating abnormal LV force.
The T axis (+50 degrees) is in the normal range.

      b. Positive voltage criteria for RVH or LVH and rela-
         tively large voltages for the other ventricle.
      c. Large equiphasic QRS complexes in two or more
         of the limb leads and in the midprecordial leads
         (V2 through V5), called Katz-Wachtel phenom-
         enon.

F. Ventricular Conduction Disturbances

    Conditions that are grouped together as ventricular con-
duction disturbances have in common abnormal prolongation of QRS duration (Fig 1-17). Ventricular conduction
disturbances and their characteristic findings include the
following:
    a. Bundle branch blocks, right and left with the pro-

longation in the terminal portion of the QRS complex (i.e., terminal slurring) (Fig 1-17, B).
b. Preexcitation (WPW syndrome) with the initial slurring or delta wave (Fig 1-17, C).
c. Intraventricular block with prolongation throughout the QRS complex (Fig 1-17, D).

The normal QRS duration varies with age (Table 1-15): in infants, a QRS duration of 0.08 sec (not 0.1 as in adults) meets the requirement for RBBB.

1. Right Bundle Branch Block

RBBB is the most common form of ventricular conduction disturbance in children. The RV depolarization is delayed and is unopposed by the LV depolarization, and therefore the terminal slow depolarization wave is directed to the right and anteriorly.

Criteria for RBBB (Fig 1-22)

a. RAD at least for terminal portion of QRS complex.
b. QRS duration longer than the upper limits of normal for the patient's age (Table 1-15).
c. Terminal slurring of the QRS complex directed to the right and usually, but not always, anteriorly.
   1) Wide and slurred S in I, V5, and V6.
   2) Terminal, slurred R′ in aVR and the RPLs (i.e., V4R, V1 and V2).
d. ST segment shift and T wave inversion are common in adults, but not in children.
e. It is unsafe to make a diagnosis of ventricular hypertrophy in the presence of RBBB. Because there is asynchrony of the opposing electromotive forces of each ventricle in RBBB, a greater manifest potential for both ventricles results.

The two most common pediatric disorders that present with RBBB are ASD and conduction disturbances following open heart surgery involving a right ventriculotomy. Other conditions often associated with RBBB include Ebstein anomaly, COA in infants less than 6 months of age, ECD, PAPVR, and occasionally in normal children. The significance of RBBB in children is different from that in

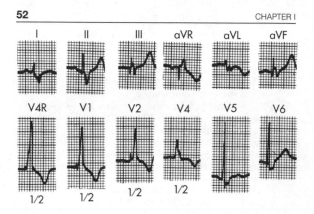

FIG. 1-22.

Tracing from a 6-year-old boy who had corrective surgery for TOF that involved right ventriculotomy for repair of VSD and resection of infundibular narrowing. The QRS axis is only minimally rightward (about +115 degrees), but the terminal (slurred) portion of the QRS is clearly rightward. The QRS duration is prolonged (0.13 sec). The T vector remains normal (+10 degrees). Although there are abnormally large R voltages in V4R, V1 and V2, with abnormal R/S ratios, one cannot be sure of RVH; it may all be due to RBBB.

adults; in many pediatric examples of RBBB, the right bundle is intact.

Although the rsR′ pattern in V1 is unusual in adults, it is normal in infants and small children provided that:

a. The QRS duration is not prolonged.
b. The voltage of the primary or secondary R waves is not abnormally large.

2. Intraventricular block
   In intraventricular block the prolongation is throughout the duration of the QRS complex (see Fig 1-17, D). It is associated with metabolic disorders (hyperkalemia), myocardial ischemia (e.g., during or after CPR), drugs (e.g., quinidine, procainamide, tricyclic

antidepressants) and diffuse myocardial diseases (myocardial fibrosis and systemic diseases with myocardial involvement).

3. Wolff-Parkinson-White syndrome

   WPW syndrome results from an anomalous conduction pathway (i.e., bundle of Kent) between the atrium and the ventricle, bypassing the normal delay of conduction in the AV node. Patients with WPW syndrome are prone to attacks of paroxysmal SVT. In the presence of this syndrome diagnosis of ventricular hypertrophy cannot be made safely, as with BBB.

   Criteria for WPW Syndrome

   a. Short PR interval, less than the lower limits of normal for the patient's age. The lower limits of normal PR interval are as follows:

      < 3 years, 0.08 sec
      3-16 years, 0.1 sec
      >16 years, 0.12 sec

   b. Delta wave (initial slurring of the QRS complex).

   c. Wide QRS duration (beyond the ULN).

      Fig 1-23 is an example of WPW syndrome.

      There are two other forms of preexcitation:

   a. Lown-Ganong-Levine syndrome is characterized by a short PR interval and normal QRS duration.

   b. Mahaim-type preexcitation is characterized by a normal PR interval and long QRS duration with a delta wave.

Ventricular Hypertrophy vs. Ventricular Conduction Disturbances

Two common pediatric ECG abnormalities, ventricular hypertrophy and ventricular conduction disturbances, are not always easy to separate. The following approach may aid in approaching an ECG for these two conditions, as well as in separating them. Fig 1-24 illustrates the general approach to the problem. An accurate measurement of the QRS duration is essential.

1. When the QRS duration is normal, normal QRS voltages indicate a normal ECG and increased QRS voltages may indicate ventricular hypertrophy.

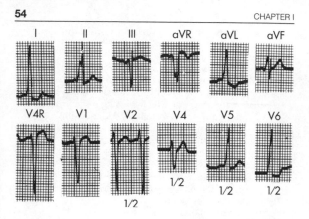

FIG. 1-23.

Tracing from a 6-month-old infant with possible glycogen storage disease. The QRS duration is increased to 0.1 sec (ULN is 0.06 for age). There are delta waves in the initial portion of the QRS complex, best seen in I, aVL, and V5. The QRS axis is 0 degree (LAD for age) and the large leftward and posterior QRS voltage are abnormal, but with preexcitation the diagnosis of LVH cannot be made.

2. When the QRS duration is clearly prolonged, normal as well as increased QRS voltages indicate ventricular conduction disturbance. An increased QRS voltage does not necessarily indicate an additional ventricular hypertrophy.

3. When the QRS duration is only borderline increased, the separation of ventricular hypertrophy and ventricular conduction disturbances is not easy. In general, a borderline increase in the QRS voltage, especially without the terminal or initial slurring, indicates probable ventricular hypertrophy rather than conduction disturbances. The slight prolongation of the QRS duration may result from a hypertrophied ventricular myocardium, which takes longer for depolarization. When the QRS voltage is normal, the ECG

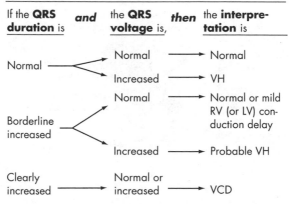

If the **QRS duration** is	*and*	the **QRS voltage** is,	*then*	the **interpretation** is
Normal		Normal		Normal
		Increased		VH
Borderline increased		Normal		Normal or mild RV (or LV) conduction delay
		Increased		Probable VH
Clearly increased		Normal or increased		VCD

FIG. 1-24.
Algorithm for differentiating between ventricular hypertrophy and ventricular conduction disturbances. VCD, ventricular conductive disturbance; VH, ventricular hypertrophy.

may be interpreted either as normal or a mild RV or LV conduction delay.

G. Pathologic ST Segment and T Wave Changes

Examples of pathologic ST segment shifts and T wave changes include LVH or RVH with strain, digitalis effects, pericarditis, including postoperative state, myocarditis and myocardial infarction.

1. Pericarditis: the ECG changes seen in pericarditis consist of the following:
   a. Pericardial effusion may produce QRS voltages less than 5 mm in every one of the limb leads.
   b. Subepicardial myocardial damage produces the following time-dependent changes in the ST segment and T wave.
      1) ST segment elevation in the leads representing the LV.

Hyperacute phase (a few hours)		Elevated ST segment Deep and wide Q wave
Early evolving phase (a few days)		Deep and wide Q wave Elevated ST segment Diphasic T wave
Late evolving phase (2-3 weeks)		Deep and wide Q wave Sharply inverted T wave
Revolving phase (for years)		Deep and wide Q wave Almost normal T wave

FIG. 1-25.
Sequential changes of ST segment and T wave in myocardial infarction. (From Park MK, Guntheroth WG: *How to read pediatric ECGs,* ed 3, St. Louis, Mosby, 1992.)

> 2) The ST segment shift returns to normal within 2 or 3 days.
> 3) T wave inversion (with isoelectric ST segment) 2 to 4 weeks after the onset of pericarditis.

2. Myocarditis: ECG findings of rheumatic or viral myocarditis are relatively nonspecific and may include the following changes which involve all phases of the cardiac cycle: first- or second-degree AV block, low QRS voltages (5 mm or less in all six limb leads), decreased amplitude of the T wave, QT prolongation, and arrhythmias.

3. Myocardial infarction: The ECG findings of myocardial infarction, which are time dependent, are illustrated in Fig 1-25. Leads that show these abnormalities vary with the location of the infarction. They are summarized in Table 1-18.

H. Electrolyte Disturbances

1. Calcium: Hypocalcemia produces the prolongation of the ST segment with resulting prolongation of the QTc interval. The T wave duration remains normal.

TABLE 1-18.

Leads Showing Abnormal ECG Findings in Myocardial Infarction

	Limb Leads	Precordial Leads
Lateral	I, aVL	V5, V6
Anterior		V1, V2, V3
Anterolateral	I, aVL	V2-V6
Diaphragmatic	II, III, aVF	

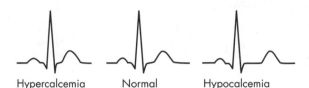

Hypercalcemia   Normal   Hypocalcemia

FIG. 1-26.

ECG findings of hypercalcemia and hypocalcemia. (From Park MK, Guntheroth WG: *How to read pediatric ECGs,* ed 3, St. Louis, Mosby, 1992.)

Hypercalcemia shortens the ST segment without affecting the T wave, with resultant shortening of the QTc interval (Fig 1-26).

2. Potassium: Hypokalemia produces one of the least specific ECG changes. When the serum potassium K level is below 2.5 mEq/L, ECG changes consist of a prominent U wave with apparent prolongation of the QTc interval, flat or diphasic T waves, and ST segment depression (Fig 1-27). With further lowering of serum K, the PR interval becomes prolonged, and sinoatrial block may occur.

A progressive hyperkalemia produces the following ECG changes (Fig 1-27): (1) tall, tented T waves, best seen in the precordial leads, (2) prolongation of QRS duration, (3) prolongation of PR interval, (4) disap-

SERUM K

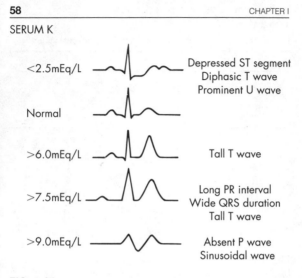

<2.5mEq/L		Depressed ST segment Diphasic T wave Prominent U wave
Normal		
>6.0mEq/L		Tall T wave
>7.5mEq/L		Long PR interval Wide QRS duration Tall T wave
>9.0mEq/L		Absent P wave Sinusoidal wave

FIG. 1-27.
ECG findings of hypokalemia and hyperkalemia. (From Park MK, Guntheroth WG: *How to read pediatric ECGs,* ed 3, St. Louis, Mosby, 1992.)

pearance of P waves, (5) wide, bizarre diphasic QRS complexes (sine wave), and (6) eventual asystole.

IV. CHEST ROENTGENOGRAPHY

Information to be gained from CXR includes (1) heart size and silhouette, (2) enlargement of specific cardiac chambers, (3) PBF or PVM, and (4) other information regarding lung parenchyma, spine, bony thorax, abdominal situs, and so on.

A. Heart Size and Silhouette

1. Heart size: The cardiothoracic (CT) ratio is obtained by dividing the largest transverse diameter of the heart with the widest internal diameter of the chest

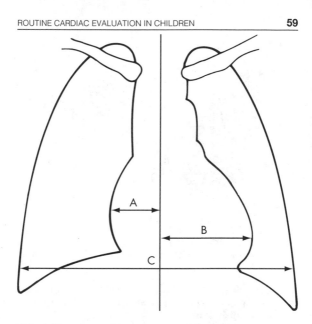

FIG. 1-28.
Measurement of the cardiothoracic (CT) ratio from the posteroanterior view of a CXR. The CT ratio is obtained by dividing the largest horizontal diameter of the heart *(A + B)* by the longest internal diameter of the chest *(C)*.

(Fig 1-28). A CT ratio of more than 0.5 is considered to indicate cardiomegaly. However, the CT ratio cannot be used with any accuracy in newborns and small infants, in whom a good inspiratory chest film is rarely obtained.

2. Normal cardiac silhouette: The structures that form the cardiac borders in the PA and lateral projections of a CXR are shown in Fig 1-29. In the newborn, however, a typical normal cardiac silhouette as shown in Fig 1-29 is rarely seen because of the presence of a

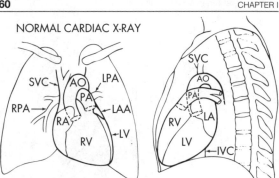

FIG. 1-29.
Posteroanterior and lateral projections of normal cardiac silhouette.
(From Park MK: *Pediatric cardiology for practitioners,* ed 3, St. Louis,
Mosby, 1995.)

> large thymus and because the MPA segment is more
> medial than in older children and does not form the
> left cardiac border.
> 3. Abnormal cardiac silhouette: The overall shape of the
>   heart sometimes provides important clues to the type
>   of defect, particularly in dealing with cyanotic patients
>   (Fig 1-30).
>   a. Boot-shaped heart with decreased PBF is seen in
>   infants with cyanotic TOF and in some infants with
>   tricuspid atresia (Fig 1-30, A).
>   b. Narrow waist and egg-shaped heart with increased
>   PBF in a cyanotic infant strongly suggests TGA (Fig
>   1-30, B).
>   c. Snowman sign with increased PBF is seen in infants
>   with the supracardiac type of TAPVR (Fig 1-30, C).

B. Cardiac Chambers and Great Arteries

> 1. Individual chamber enlargement
>   a. LAE—Mild LAE is best recognized in the lateral

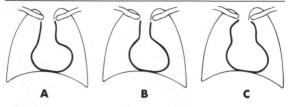

FIG. 1-30.
Abnormal cardiac silhouette. **A,** boot-shaped heart. **B,** egg-shaped heart. **C,** snowman sign. (From Park MK: *Pediatric cardiology for practitioners,* ed 3, St. Louis, Mosby, 1995.)

    projection by posterior protrusion of the LA border. An enlargement of the LA may produce a double density on the PA view. With further enlargement the left atrial appendage becomes prominent on the left cardiac border and the left main-stem bronchus is elevated.

   b. LVE,—in the PA view the apex of the heart is displaced to the left and inferiorly. In the lateral view the lower posterior cardiac border is displaced further posteriorly.

   c. RAE, in the PA projection an enlargement of the RA results in an increased prominence of the right lower cardiac border.

   d. RVE is best recognized in the lateral view by the filling of the retrosternal space.

2. The size of the great arteries

   a. Prominent MPA segment: Prominence of a normally placed pulmonary artery (PA) in the PA view (Fig 1-31, A) is due to one of the following:

     1) Poststenotic dilatation (e.g., pulmonary valve stenosis).

     2) Increased blood flow through the PA (e.g., ASD, VSD).

     3) Increased pressure in the PA (i.e., pulmonary hypertension).

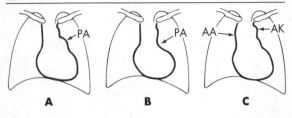

FIG. 1-31.
Abnormalities of the great arteries. **A,** prominent main PA segment.
B, concave PA segment. **C,** dilation of the ascending aorta *(AA)* and
a prominence of the aortic knob *(AK)*. (From Park MK: *Pediatric
cardiology for practitioners,* ed 3, St. Louis, Mosby, 1995.)

      4) Occasional normal adolescence, especially in
         girls.
  b. A concave MPA segment with resulting boot-
     shaped heart is seen in TOF and tricuspid atresia
     (Fig 1-31, B).
  c. Dilatation of the aorta. An enlarged ascending
     aorta (AA) is seen in AS (poststenotic dilatation)
     and TOF and less often in PDA, COA, or systemic
     hypertension. When the ascending aorta and
     aortic arch are enlarged, the aortic knob (AK) may
     become prominent on the PA view (Fig 1-31, C).

C. Pulmonary Vascular Markings

One of the major goals of radiologic examination is the
assessment of the pulmonary vasculature.
1. Increased PVM is present when the pulmonary arteries appear enlarged and extend into the lateral third
of the lung field, where they are not usually present,
and there is an increased vascularity to the lung
apices where the vessels are normally collapsed.
    Increased PVM in an acyanotic child reflects ASD,
VSD, PDA, ECD, PAPVR, or any combination of these.
In a cyanotic infant, an increased PVM may indicate
TGA, TAPVR, HLHS, persistent truncus arteriosus, or
single ventricle.

2. A decreased PVM is suspected when the hilum appears small, the remaining lung fields appear black, and the vessels appear small and thin. Ischemic lung fields in cyanotic patients suggest critical stenosis or atresia of the pulmonary or tricuspid valves or TOF.

3. Pulmonary venous congestion, which is characterized by a hazy and indistinct margin of the pulmonary vasculature, is seen with HLHS, MS, TAPVR, cor triatriatum, and so on.

4. Normal pulmonary vasculature is present in patients with mild to moderate obstructive lesions (e.g., PS or AS) and in patients with small L-R shunt lesions.

D. Systematic Approach

The interpretation of CXRs should include a systematic routine to avoid overlooking important anatomic changes relevant to cardiac diagnosis.

1. Location of the liver and stomach gas bubble: The cardiac apex should be on the same side as the stomach or opposite the hepatic shadow. When there is heterotaxia, with the apex on the right and the stomach on the left, or vice versa, the likelihood of serious heart defect is great. A midline liver is associated with asplenia (Ivemark) syndrome or polysplenia syndrome.

2. Skeletal aspect of CXR: Pectus excavatum may create the false impression of cardiomegaly in the PA projection. Thoracic scoliosis and vertebral abnormalities are frequent findings in cardiac patients. Rib notching is a specific finding of COA in a child usually older than 5 years, generally between the fourth and eighth ribs.

3. Identification of the aorta: When the descending aorta is seen on the left vertebral column, a left aortic arch is present. When the descending aorta is seen on the right of the vertebral column, a right arch is present. A right aortic arch is frequently associated with TOF or persistent truncus arteriosus. A figure 3 in a heavily exposed film or an E-shaped indentation in a barium esophagogram is seen with COA.

4. Upper mediastinum: The thymus is prominent in healthy infants and may give a false impression of cardiomegaly. A narrow mediastinal shadow is seen in TGA or DiGeorge syndrome. A snowman figure (figure 8 configuration) is seen in infants (usually older than 4 months) with supracardiac TAPVR.

5. Pulmonary parenchyma: A longstanding density, particularly in the right lower lung field, suggests bronchopulmonary sequestration. A vertical vascular shadow along the right lower cardiac border may suggest PAPVR from the lower lobe (the scimitar syndrome).

TABLE 1-19.

Flow Diagram of Congenital Heart Disease

Acyanotic Defects	
Increased PBF	
LVH or CVH	VSD, PDA, ECD
RVH	ASD (often RBBB), PAPVR, Eisenmenger physiology (secondary to VSD, PDA, and so on)
Normal PBF	
LVH	AS or AR, COA, endocardial fibroelastosis, MR
RVH	PS, COA in infants, MS
Cyanotic Defects	
Increased PBF	
LVH or CVH	Persistent truncus arteriosus, single ventricle, TGA + VSD
RVH	TGA, TAPVR, HLHS
Decreased PBF	
CVH	TGA + PS, Truncus with hypoplastic PA, single ventricle + PS
LVH	Tricuspid atresia, pulmonary atresia with hypoplastic RV
RVH	TOF, Eisenmenger physiology (secondary to ASD, VSD, PDA), Ebstein anomaly (RBBB)

V. FLOW DIAGRAM

A flow diagram that often helps in arriving at a diagnosis of CHD is shown in Table 1-19. It is based on the presence or absence of cyanosis and the status of PBF. Ventricular hypertrophy on the ECG further narrows down the possibilities. Only common entities are listed in the flow diagram.

SPECIAL TOOLS IN CARDIAC EVALUATION

I. ECHOCARDIOGRAPHY

A. M-Mode Echocardiography

The M-mode echo, which provides an "ice pick" view of the heart, is important in the evaluation of certain cardiac conditions and functions, particularly in the measurement of dimensions and timing. An M-mode echo through three important structures of the left side of the heart is illustrated in Fig 2-1.

1. Applications of the M-mode echo
   a. Measurement of the dimensions of cardiac chambers and vessels and the thickness of the ventricular septum and free walls.
   b. LV systolic function (e.g., fractional shortening, ejection fraction).
   c. Study of the motion of valves (e.g., MVP, MS, pulmonary hypertension) and the interventricular septum.
   d. Detection of pericardial fluid.
2. Normal M-mode echo values (See Appendix, Tables A-3, A-4)
3. LV Function (see Table A-4)
   a. Fractional shortening (FS) of the LV is as follows:

$$FS\ (\%) = \frac{Dd - Ds}{Dd} \times 100,$$

   where Dd is end-diastolic dimension and Ds is end-systolic dimension.

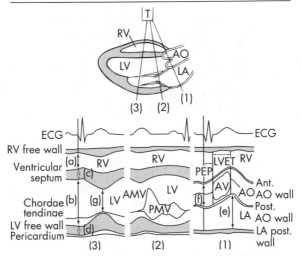

FIG. 2-1.
Cross-sectional view of the left side of the heart along the long axis
(top) through which ice pick views of the M-mode echo recordings
are made *(bottom)*. a, RV dimension. b, LV diastolic dimension (Dd).
c, thickness of ventricular septum. d, thickness of posterior free wall.
e, LA dimension. f, aortic dimension. g, LV systolic dimension (Ds).
AMV, anterior mitral valve. *PMV,* posterior mitral valve. *LVET,* LV
ejection time. *PEP,* pre-ejection period. (From Park MK: *Pediatric
Cardiology for Practitioners,* ed 3. St. Louis, Mosby, 1995.)

Normal FS is 36% (28% to 44%, 95% CI).
b. Ejection fraction (EF) is obtained by this formula:

$$EF\ (\%) = \frac{(Dd)^3 - (Ds)^3}{(Dd)^3} \times 100.$$

Normal EF is 74% (64% to 83%, 95% CI).
c. Systolic time intervals

The preejection period (PEP) reflects the rate of pressure rise in the ventricle during isovolumic systole. The ratio of PEP to the ventricular ejection time (PEP/VET) is little affected by changes in heart rate. The method of measuring LPEP and LVET is shown in Figure 2-1. Normal values (and ranges) for the RV and LV are as follows:

RPEP/RVET, 0.24 (0.16 to 0.3)
LPEP/LVET, 0.35 (0.3 to 0.39)

B. Two-Dimensional Echo

The 2D echo better demonstrates the spatial relationship of structures and therefore provides a more accurate anatomic diagnosis of abnormalities of the heart and great vessels. Routine 2D echo is obtained from four transducer locations: parasternal, apical, subcostal, and suprasternal notch positions. Figs 2-2 through 2-5 illustrate selected standard images of the heart and great vessels. Selected normal values are presented in the Appendix, Tables A-5 and A-6.

C. Color Flow Mapping

A color-coded Doppler provides images of the direction and disturbances of blood flow superimposed on the echo structural image. The red flows toward and the blue flows away from the transducer. A turbulent flow appears as light green. This is useful in the detection of shunt or valvular lesions.

D. Doppler Echo

Doppler ultrasound equipment detects frequency shifts and thus determines the direction and velocity of blood flow with respect to the ultrasound beam. The pulsed wave (PW) Doppler can control the site at which Doppler signals are sampled, but the maximum detectable velocity is limited so that it cannot be used for quantification of severe obstruction. On the other hand, the continuous wave (CW) Doppler can measure very high velocities for the estimation of severe stenosis. A positive Doppler indicates a flow toward the transducer, and a negative Doppler, a flow away from it.

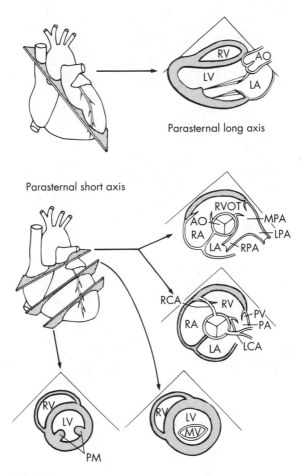

FIG. 2-2.
Important 2D echo views obtained from the parasternal transducer position. (From Park MK. *Pediatric Cardiology for Practitioners,* ed 3. St. Louis, Mosby, 1995.)

Apical views

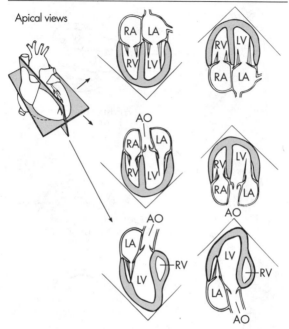

FIG. 2-3.
2D echo views obtained with the tranducer at the apical position.
Both the apex-down and apex-up images are shown. (From Park
MK. *Pediatric Cardiology for Practitioners,* ed 3. St. Louis, Mosby,
1995.)

An estimation of pressure gradient $(P_1 - P_2)$ can be
obtained by a modified Bernoulli equation:

$$P_1 - P_2 = 4(V2^2 - V1^2) = 4V^2,$$

where V2 is peak Doppler velocity beyond the obstruction
and V1 is peak Doppler velocity proximal to the obstruction.

Subcostal views

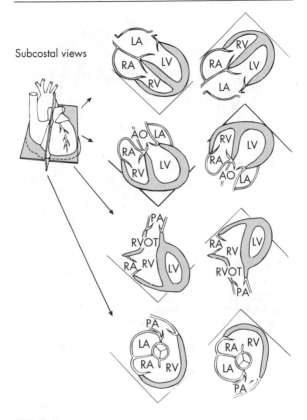

FIG. 2-4.
2D echo views obtained with the transducer at the subcostal position. Both the apex-down and apex-up images are shown. (From Park MK. *Pediatric Cardiology for Practitioners,* ed 3. St. Louis, Mosby, 1995.)

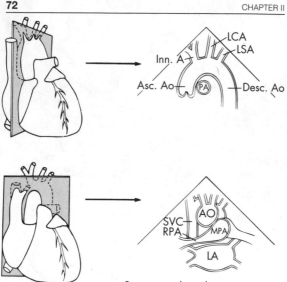

FIG. 2-5.
Suprasternal notch 2D echo views. *Asc. Ao,* ascending aorta. *Desc. Ao,* descending aorta. *Inn. A,* innominate artery. *LCA,* left carotid artery. *LSA,* left subclavian artery. (From Park MK. *Pediatric Cardiology for Practitioners,* ed 3. St. Louis, Mosby, 1995)

With this formula the severity of AS, PS, or COA can be estimated. Pressures in the RV can also be estimated from the flow velocity of a TR or through a VSD. For example, if the maximum flow velocity through the aortic valve is 4 m/sec, a transaortic (instantaneous) systolic pressure gradient is 64 mm Hg ($4^2 \times 4 = 64$). If the TR velocity is 3 m/sec, the RV systolic pressure is estimated to be about 41 mm Hg. This is derived from $3^2 \times 4 = 36$ mm Hg plus the estimated RA pressure of 5 mm Hg.

In patients with COA an accurate pressure gradient is obtained by using the maximum flow velocity proximal to

(V1) and distal to (V2) the coarctation. For example, if the V1 if 1.6 m/sec and the V2 is 3.2 m/sec, the transcoarctation gradient is 30 mm Hg. This is derived from

$$4 \times (3.2^2 - 1.6^2) = 4 \times (10.2 - 2.6) = 4 \times 7.5 = 30 \text{ mm Hg}$$

II. EXERCISE TEST

Exercise testing is important in evaluating cardiac symptoms and arrhythmias, quantifying the severity of the cardiac abnormality, and assessing the effectiveness of management. Stress testing has been found to be useful in evaluating the following cardiac conditions in children:

1. AS: Ischemic changes on the ECG during exercise may be an indication for surgical intervention, regardless of predicted pressure gradients.
2. AR: Patients who develop ST segment changes or fail to raise their heart rate with exercise may have LV dysfunction and may need surgical valve replacement.
3. Arrhythmias: Ventricular arrhythmias increasing in frequency with exercise may require therapy. The efficacy of antiarrhythmic therapy can also be evaluated by exercise testing. If ventricular arrhythmias are abolished by exercise and not associated with organic cardiac disorders, they can generally be ignored.
4. AV block: AV blocks that worsen with exercise warrant therapy.
5. Postoperative evaluation of TOF and other cyanotic CHD: a patient who develops multiform PVCs or ventricular tachycardia may be a candidate for sudden death and requires either antiarrhythmic therapy or surgical intervention.
6. Postcoarctectomy patients: patients who develop an excessive increase in blood pressure with exercise may need antihypertensive measures.
7. Rarely, adolescents with chest pain may need stress testing to rule out cardiac cause.
8. Appropriate exercise prescription for participation in vocational, recreational, and competitive activities.

Treadmill protocols are well standardized and more widely used than bicycle ergometer protocol. Normal values for children are available for the Bruce protocol. Endurance time appears to be the best predictor of exercise capacity in children by the Bruce protocol (Table 2-1). During stress testing the patient is continuously monitored for ischemic changes or arrhythmias by ECG, symptoms such as chest pain or faintness, heart rate responses (normal 190 to 200 beats/min) and blood pressure response (normal systolic pressures may rise to 180 mm Hg).

III. AMBULATORY ELECTROCARDIOGRAPHY

Ambulatory ECG monitoring is useful in the diagnosis of arrhythmias that are likely to occur but are not revealed by a routine ECG. Adhesive ECG electrodes are attached to the chest wall, and an ECG rhythm is continually registered for 24 hours or longer by using a small, battery-driven cassette tape recorder (i.e., Holter monitor). It has a built-in timer used in conjunction with the patient's diary to allow subsequent correlation of the patient's symptoms and activities with arrhythmias. The tape is played back on a high-speed data analysis system and analyzed by a computerized arrhythmia-detection template. Events of interest can be picked out and printed for review and record.

Ambulatory ECG monitoring is obtained for the following reasons:

1. To determine whether symptoms such as chest pain, palpitation, or syncope were caused by cardiac arrhythmias.
2. To evaluate the adequacy of medical therapy for an arrhythmia.
3. To screen high-risk cardiac patients, such as those with hypertrophic cardiomyopathy or those who had surgical operations known to predispose to arrhythmias (Mustard, Senning, Fontan-type operations).
4. To evaluate possible intermittent pacemaker failure.
5. To determine the effect of sleep on potentially life-threatening arrhythmias.

The Holter recordings should reveal the frequency, duration, and types of arrhythmias, as well as precipitating or terminating events of arrhythmias. In children significant arrhythmias are infrequently the cause of symptoms such as palpitation, chest pain, and syncope (fewer than 10% of

TABLE 2-1.

Bruce Treadmill Test Endurance Times (min)

Age (yr)	Percentile						Mean	SD
	10	25	50	75	90			
Boys								
4-5	8.1	9.0	10.0	12.0	13.3		10.4	1.9
6-7	9.7	10.0	12.0	12.3	13.5		11.8	1.6
8-9	9.6	10.5	12.4	13.7	16.2		12.6	2.3
10-12	9.9	12.0	12.5	14.0	15.4		12.7	1.9
13-15	11.2	13.0	14.3	16.0	16.1		14.1	1.7
16-18	11.3	12.1	13.6	14.5	15.8		13.5	1.4
Girls								
4-5	7.0	8.0	9.0	11.2	12.3		9.5	1.8
6-7	9.5	9.6	11.4	13.0	13.0		11.2	1.5
8-9	9.9	10.5	11.0	13.0	14.2		11.8	1.6
10-12	10.5	11.3	12.0	13.0	14.6		12.3	1.4
13-15	9.4	10.0	11.5	12.0	13.0		11.1	1.3
16-18	8.1	10.0	10.5	12.0	12.4		10.7	1.4

Adapted from Cumming GR, Everatt D, Hastman L: Am J Cardiol 41:69-75, 1978.

cases). Marked bradycardia (below 50 beats/min in infants or 40 beats/min in older children), SVT with rate over 200 beats/min, or ventricular tachycardia may be life threatening. These arrhythmias may worsen during sleep. Ambulatory ECG monitoring is not very helpful in detecting an episode that occurs infrequently (i.e., once a week or once a month) and is unnecessary for asymptomatic extrasystoles.

IV. CARDIAC CATHETERIZATION AND ANGIOCARDIOGRAPHY

Cardiac catheterization and angiocardiography are the definitive diagnostic tests for most cardiac patients. They are carried out under any of various general sedatives (see section B). For newborns, cyanotic infants, and hemodynamically unstable children, general anesthesia with intubation may be employed.

A. Indications

Indications for these invasive studies vary from institution to institution and from cardiologist to cardiologist. With improved capability of noninvasive techniques (2D echo and color flow Doppler studies), many cardiac problems are adequately diagnosed and managed without the invasive studies. The following are considered indications by most but not all cardiologists.

1. Selected newborns with cyanotic CHD who may require palliative surgery or balloon atrial septostomy during the procedure.
2. Selected children with CHD when the lesion is severe enough to require surgical intervention.
3. Children who appear to have had unsatisfactory results from cardiac surgery.
4. Infants and children with lesions amenable to balloon angioplasty or valvuloplasty.

B. Sedation

Various sedatives alone or in combination have been used by different institutions with equally good success rates. In general, smaller doses of sedatives are used in cyanotic infants.

1. No sedation is used in the newborn.
2. For infants less than 10 kg, a combination of chloral hydrate 75 mg/kg, maximum 2 g PO and diphenhydramine 2 mg/kg, maximum 100 mg PO has been used with good results.
3. For older children, Demerol compound, a solution containing 25 mg/ml of meperidine (Demerol), 12.5 mg/ml of promethazine (Phenergan) and 12.5 mg/ml of chloropromazine (Thorazine), is popular. The dose of the Demerol compound is 0.11 ml/kg IM. Some centers exclude chloropromazine from the mixture. In cyanotic children the dose is reduced by one-third. For children with severe CHF the dose is reduced by half.
4. A combination of meperidine 1 mg/kg and hydroxyzine (Vistaril) 1 m/kg IM or a combination of fentanyl 1.25 mg/kg and droperidol 62.5 mg/kg IM gives an equally good result.
5. Ketamine 3 mg/kg IM or 1 to 2 mg/kg IV may be used, but it can change the hemodynamic data because it increases the systemic vascular resistance and blood pressure.
6. Morphine 0.1 to 0.2 mg/kg administered subcutaneously has been used to prevent or treat hypoxic spells in cyanotic infants.
7. If more sedation is required during the study, intravenous diazepam (Valium) 0.1 mg/kg or morphine 0.1 mg/kg is used.

C. Normal Hemodynamic Values and Their Calculations

Pressure and oxygen saturation values for normal children are shown in Fig 2-6. Cardiac output, cardiac shunt, and vascular resistance are routinely calculated.

1. Flows (cardiac output) are calculated by the Fick formula:

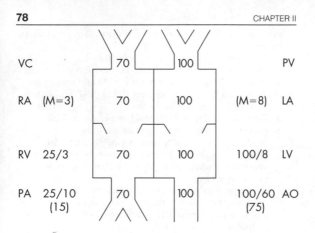

FIG. 2-6.
Pressure and oxygen saturation values in normal children.

$$\text{Pulmonary flow (Qp)} = \frac{VO_2}{C_{PV} - C_{PA}}$$

$$\text{Systemic flow (Qs)} = \frac{VO_2}{C_{AO} - C_{MV}}$$

where flows are in liters per minute, VO_2 is oxygen consumption in milliliters per minute, C is oxygen content in milliliters per liter at various positions, PV is the pulmonary vein, PA is the pulmonary artery, AO is the aorta, and MV is mixed systemic venous blood (SVC or RA).

Oxygen consumption is either directly measured during the procedure or estimated from a table (see Appendix, Table A-7). Oxygen content (milliliters per 100 ml) is derived by multiplying oxygen capacity by percent saturation. Oxygen capacity (milliliters per 100 ml) is the total content of oxygen that hemoglobin contains when it is 100% saturated ($1.36 \times$ hemoglobin in grams per 100 ml). Normal systemic flow (or pulmonary flow in the absence of shunt) is 3.1 ± 0.4 L/min/m^2 (i.e., cardiac index).

2. The magnitude of the shunt is calculated as follows:

$$\text{L-R shunt} = Qp - Qs$$
$$\text{R-L shunt} = Qs - Qp$$

In pediatrics the ratio of pulmonary to systemic flow (Qp/Qs), which does not require an oxygen consumption value, is often used. The ratio provides information on the magnitude of the shunt. Patients with an L-R shunt greater than 2:1 are usually candidates for surgery.

3. Vascular resistances are calculated by using formulas derived from Ohm's law ($R = \Delta P/Q$).

$$PVR = \frac{\text{Mean PA pressure} - \text{mean LA pressure}}{Qp}$$

$$SVR = \frac{\text{Mean aortic pressure} - \text{mean RA pressure}}{Qs}$$

The normal SVR varies between 15 and 30 units/m^2. The normal PVR is high at birth but reaches near-adult values (1 to 3 units/m^2) after 2 to 4 months. Normal ratio of PVR/SVR ranges from 1:20 to 1:10.

D. Selective Angiocardiography

A radiopaque dye is rapidly injected through a cardiac catheter into a certain site and angiograms are recorded on motion picture film at 60 or 90 frames per second, often on biplane views. The dose of angiographic dyes for an angiogram ranges from 1 to 2 ml/kg of body weight, depending on the nature of the defect. Nonionizing contrast media with low osmolality (e.g., Isovue, Omnipaque) are widely used because of their low incidence of side effects.

E. Risks

Cardiac catheterization and angiocardiography can lead to serious complications, including (rarely) death. Complications include serious arrhythmias, heart block, cardiac perforation, hypoxic spells, arterial obstruction, hemorrhage, infection, reactions to the contrast material, intramyocardial injection of the contrast, and renal complications (hematuria, proteinuria, oliguria, anuria). Hypothermia, acidemia, hypoglycemia, convulsions, hypotension, and respiratory depression are more likely in the newborn infant.

In general, the risk of cardiac catheterization and angiocardiography varies with the age and illness of the patient, the type of lesion, and the experience of those doing the procedure. The reported rate of fatal complications varies from less than 1% to as high as 5% in newborns. About 3% to 5% of patients have significant nonfatal complications such as arrhythmias and arterial complications. However, careful preparation and monitoring and the use of prostaglandin infusion in selected newborns can keep the mortality and morbidity to a minimum.

F. Preparation and Monitoring

Adequate preparation of the patient and careful monitoring during the procedure can minimize complications and fatality from the invasive studies. The following areas are particularly important.

1. Increasing temperature in the cardiac catheterization laboratory, using a warming blanket, and monitoring rectal temperature to avoid hypothermia when an infant is being studied.
2. Monitoring oxygen saturation transcutaneously, checking arterial blood gases and pH, and correcting acidemia and hypoxemia; correcting hypoglycemia or hypocalcemia before the start of the procedure.
3. Monitoring oxygen saturation and administering oxygen, if indicated, during the procedure.
4. Intubating or readiness for intubating in infants with respiratory difficulties, and having emergency medications (e.g., atropine, epinephrine, bicarbonate) drawn up and ready.
5. Initiating prostaglandin infusion in cyanotic infants who appear to be ductus dependent.
6. Whenever possible, having another physician or an anesthesiologist available to monitor noncardiac aspects of the patient.

CONGENITAL HEART DEFECTS

III

I. LEFT-TO-RIGHT SHUNT LESIONS

A. Atrial Septal Defect (Ostium Secundum ASD)

Prevalence: 5% to 10% of all CHD

Pathology and Pathophysiology

1. Three types of ASD occur in the atrial septum. Secundum ASD is in the central portion of the septum and is the most common type (50% to 70% of ASDs). Primum ASD, (or partial ECD), in the lower part of the septum (30% of ASDs). Sinus venosus defect is near the entrance of the SVC or IVC to the RA (about 10% of all ASDs). PAPVR is common with a sinus venous defect. MVP is occasionally associated with the secundum type or a sinus venosus ASD.

2. An L-R shunt is present through the defect with a volume overload to the RA and RV and an increase in pulmonary blood flow. Pulmonary hypertension usually develops in adult life.

Clinical Manifestations

1. The patients are usually asymptomatic.

2. A relatively slender body build is typical. A widely split and fixed S2 and a grade 2 to 3/6 systolic ejection murmur at the ULSB are characteristic. With a large L-R shunt, a middiastolic rumble (resulting from relative TS) may be audible at the LLSB.

3. The ECG shows RAD (+90 to +180) and mild RVH or RBBB with an rsR' pattern in V1.

4. CXR films show cardiomegaly (with RAE and RVE), increased PVM, and a prominent MPA segment.

5. 2D echo shows the position as well as the size of the defect. Cardiac catheterization is usually not necessary.

6. Spontaneous closure of the defect occurs in the first 4 years of life in about 40% of patients. With small defects the spontaneous closure rate is very high, over 80%, in the first 18 months of life. The defect may shrink in some patients. If the defect is large and left untreated, pulmonary hypertension, CHF, and atrial arrhythmias may occur in the third and fourth decades of adult life. Cerebrovascular accident due to paradoxic embolization through an ASD is possible.

Management

Medical: Exercise restriction is not required. Subacute bacterial endocarditis (SBE) prophylaxis is not indicated unless MVP or PAPVR is associated with the defect. Various devices for nonsurgical closure of the defect using cardiac catheters are in an experimental stage.

Surgical: Open repair (simple suture or with a patch) under cardiopulmonary bypass is performed when the patient is 3 to 5 years old, with surgical mortality less than 1%. An L-R shunt with a Qp/Qs of 1.5:1 or greater is an indication for surgery. Some recommend closure of even smaller defects because of the risk of a paradoxic embolization and CVA. High PVR (≥ 10 units/m^2) is a contraindication to surgery.

Postsurgical: Atrial or nodal arrhythmias occur in 7% to 20% of patients. Occasional sick sinus syndrome requires pacemaker therapy.

B. Ventricular Septal Defect

Prevalence: VSD is the most common form of CHD, (20% to 25% of CHDs except those occurring as part of cyanotic CHD).

Pathology and Pathophysiology

1. The ventricular septum consists of a small membranous septum and a larger muscular septum. The muscular septum consists of the inlet, infundibular,

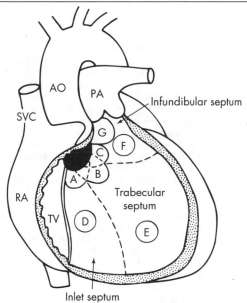

FIG. 3-1.
Anatomic locations of various VSDs, viewed with the RV free wall removed. Black area is the membranous ventricular septum. *A,* perimembranous inlet ("AV canal–type") VSD; *B,* perimembranous trabecular (typical membranous) VSD; *C,* perimembranous infundibular ("tetralogy-type") VSD; *D,* inlet muscular VSD; *E,* trabecular muscular VSD; *F,* infundibular or outlet muscular VSD; *G,* subarterial infundibular (supracristal) VSD.

and trabecular (or simply muscular) septum (Fig 3-1). A membranous VSD often involves a varying amount of muscular septum adjacent to it (i.e., perimembranous VSD). The perimembranous defect is more common (70%) than the trabecular (5% to 20%), infundibular, or inlet defects. PDA and COA are frequently associated with it. In subarterial infundibular or supracristal VSD the aortic valve may prolapse through the VSD, with resulting AR.

2. The defect varies in size from small and without hemodynamic significance to a large defect with pulmonary hypertension and CHF. In VSDs with small to moderate L-R shunts, volume overload is placed on the LA and LV but not on the RV. With larger defects the RV is under volume and pressure overload in addition to a greater volume overload on the LA and LV. PBF is increased to a varying degree, and pulmonary hypertension may result. With a long-standing large VSD, PVOD develops, with severe pulmonary hypertension and cyanosis resulting from an R-L shunt.

Clinical Manifestations

1. Patients with small VSDs are asymptomatic, with normal growth and development. With moderate to large VSDs delayed growth and development, repeated pulmonary infections, CHF, and decreased exercise tolerance are relatively common. With PVOD cyanosis and a decreased level of activity may result.

2. A grade 2 to 5/6 regurgitant systolic murmur (holosystolic or less than holosystolic) maximally audible at the LLSB is characteristic. A systolic thrill may be present at the LLSB. An apical diastolic rumble is an indication of a large L-R shunt through the defect. The S2 may split narrowly, and the intensity of the P2 increases if pulmonary hypertension is present.

3. ECG findings: Small VSD, normal; Moderate VSD, LVH, LAH (±); Large VSD, CVH and LAH (±); PVOD, pure RVH.

4. CXR films reveal cardiomegaly of varying degrees with enlargement of the LA, LV, and possibly the RV. PVMs are increased. The degree of cardiomegaly and the increase in PVMs are directly related to the magnitude of the L-R shunt. In PVOD the MPA and the hilar pulmonary arteries are notably enlarged, but the peripheral lung fields are ischemic.

5. 2D echo studies provide accurate diagnosis of the position and size of the VSD. LA and LV dimensions provide indirect assessment of the magnitude of the shunt. The Doppler studies of the PA, TR if present, and the VSD itself are useful in indirect assessment of RV and PA pressures.

6. Spontaneous closure occurs in 30% to 40% of all VSDs, most often in small trabecular VSDs, more frequently in small defects than in large defects, and more often in the first year of life than thereafter. Large defects tend to become smaller with age. Inlet and infundibular VSDs do not become smaller or close spontaneously. CHF develops in infants with a large VSD but usually not until 6 or 8 weeks of age. PVOD may begin to develop as early as 6 to 12 months of age in patients with a large VSD, but an R-L shunt is rare before the second decade of life. Infective endocarditis is uncommon.

Management

Medical: Treatment of CHF with digitalis and diuretics (see Chapter 7). No exercise restriction is required in the absence of pulmonary hypertension. Maintenance of good dental hygiene and prophylaxis against SBE are important.

Surgical

a. Procedure
   1) PA banding as a palliative procedure is rarely performed unless additional lesions make the complete repair difficult.
   2) Direct closure of the defect is performed under cardiopulmonary bypass and/or deep hypothermia, preferably through an atrial approach rather than through a right ventriculotomy.

b. Indications and timing
   1) A significant L-R shunt with a Qp/Qs of greater than 2:1 is an indication for surgical closure. Surgery is not indicated for a small VSD with Qp/Qs less than 1.5:1.
   2) Infants with CHF and growth retardation unresponsive to medical therapy should be operated

on at any age, including early infancy. Infants
with a large VSD and evidence of increasing
PVR should be operated on as soon as possible.
Infants who respond to medical therapy may
be operated on by the age of 12 to 18 months.
Asymptomatic children may be operated on between 2 and 4 years of age.
   3) Contraindications: PVR/SVR ratio 0.5 or greater
   or PVOD with a predominant R-L shunt.
   c. Surgical approaches for special situations
      1) VSD + PDA: If PDA is large, the ductus alone
      may be closed in the first 6 to 8 weeks, and the
      VSD may be closed later.
      2) VSD + COA: Controversies exist. One approach
      is the repair of COA alone initially without PA
      banding. The VSD is closed later if indicated.
      3) VSD + AR is usually associated with subarterial
      infundibular (or supracristal) VSD and occa-
      sionally with perimembranous VSD. When AR is
      present, a prompt closure of the VSD is recom-
      mended, even if the Qp/Qs is less than 2:1, to
      abort progression of or to abolish AR. When AR
      is moderate or severe, the aortic valve is
      repaired or replaced.
   Postsurgical Follow-up: No restriction in activity unless complications have resulted from surgery. SBE
   prophylaxis may be discontinued 6 months after the
   surgery when no residual shunt is present. If a
   residual shunt is present, SBE prophylaxis should
   be observed.

C. Patent Ductus Arteriosus

   Prevalence: 5% to 10% of all CHDs, excluding those in
   premature infants.
   Pathology and Pathophysiology
   1. There is a persistent patency of a normal fetal structure between the PA and the descending aorta.
   2. The magnitude of the L-R shunt is determined by the
   diameter and length of the ductus and the level of
   PVR. With a long-standing large ductus, pulmonary

hypertension and PVOD may develop with an R-L shunt and cyanosis.

Clinical Manifestations

1. Asymptomatic when the ductus is small. When the defect is large, CHF may develop.

2. A grade 1 to 4/6 continuous (machinery) murmur best audible at the ULSB or left infraclavicular area is the hallmark of the condition. An apical diastolic rumble is audible with a large-shunt PDA. Bounding peripheral pulses with wide pulse pressure are present with a large-shunt PDA.

3. ECG findings are similar to those of VSD: Normal or LVH in a small to moderate PDA; CVH in a large PDA; RVH if PVOD develops.

4. CXR findings are also similar to those of VSD: Normal with a small-shunt PDA. With a large-shunt PDA, cardiomegaly (with LAE and LVE) and increased PVM are present. With PVOD the heart size is normal, with a marked prominence of the MPA and hilar vessels.

5. The PDA can be directly imaged and its hemodynamic significance determined by 2D echo and color flow Doppler examination. Cardiac catheterization is usually not indicated in isolated PDA.

6. CHF or recurrent pneumonia or both develop if the shunt is large. Spontaneous closure of PDA usually does not occur in term infants. PVOD may develop if a large PDA with pulmonary hypertension is left untreated.

Management

   Medical: No exercise restriction is required in the absence of pulmonary hypertension. Indomethacin is ineffective in term infants with PDA. SBE prophylaxis should be observed when indications arise. Catheter closure of PDA with various devices has been reported.

   Surgical: Ligation and division through left posterolateral thoracotomy without cardiopulmonary bypass is indicated for all PDAs regardless of size. Surgical mortality is less than 1%. PVOD is a contraindication to surgery.

Postsurgical: No restriction of activity is indicated unless pulmonary hypertension persists. SBE prophylaxis is not indicated beyond 6 months after successful surgery.

Differential Diagnosis: The following are the conditions that may present with continuous murmurs:

1. Coronary AV fistula (the murmur is audible over the precordium, not maximally at the ULSB).
2. Systemic AV fistula (a wide pulse pressure with bounding pulse, CHF, and a continuous murmur over the fistula (head or liver) are characteristic).
3. Pulmonary AV fistula (a continuous murmur over the back, cyanosis, and clubbing in the absence of cardiomegaly).
4. Venous hum (disappears when the patient is supine).
5. Murmurs of collaterals in patients with COA or TOF (audible in the intercostal spaces).
6. VSD + AR (maximally audible at the MLSB or LLSB, it is actually a to-and-fro murmur, rather than a continuous murmur).
7. Absence of pulmonary valve (a to-and-fro murmur, or "sawing-wood sound" at the ULSB, large central pulmonary arteries on the CXR film, RVH on the ECG, and cyanosis).
8. Persistent truncus arteriosus occasionally.
9. Aortopulmonary septal defect (AP window).
10. Peripheral PA stenosis (a continuous murmur may be audible all over the thorax, unilateral or bilateral).
11. Ruptured sinus of Valsalva aneurysm (sudden onset of severe heart failure is characteristic).
12. TAPVR draining into the RA (best audible along the right sternal border).
13. Obstruction to pulmonary venous return following the Mustard operation for TGA (along the right sternal border).

D. Complete Endocardial Cushion Defect (Complete AV Canal)

Prevalence: 2% of all CHD. 30% of the defects occur in children with Down syndrome. Some 40% of children

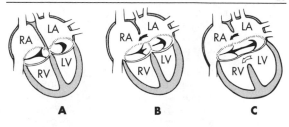

FIG. 3-2.

AV valve and cardiac septa in partial and complete ECDs. **A,** Normal AV valve anatomy with no septal defects. **B,** Partial ECD with clefts in the mitral and tricuspid valves and an ostium primum ASD *(arrow)*. **C,** Complete ECD. There is a common AV valve with large anterior and posterior bridging leaflets. An ostium primum ASD *(solid arrow)* and an inlet VSD *(open arrow)* are present.

with Down syndrome have CHDs, and 40% of the defects are ECD.

Pathology and Pathophysiology

1. Complete ECD consists of ostium primum ASD, VSD in the inlet portion of the ventricular septum, a cleft in the anterior mitral valve leaflet, and a cleft in the septal leaflet of the tricuspid valve, together with the cleft mitral valve, forming common anterior and posterior cusps of the AV valve (Fig 3-2). When the ventricular septum is intact, the defect is termed partial ECD or ostium primum ASD.

2. The combination of these defects may result in an interatrial and/or interventricular shunt, LV-to-RA shunt, or AV valve regurgitation. CHF with or without pulmonary hypertension usually develops early in infancy.

Clinical Manifestations

1. Failure to thrive, repeated respiratory infections, and signs of CHF are common.

2. Hyperactive precordium with a systolic thrill at the LLSB and a loud S2 are frequent findings. A grade 3 to 4/6 holosystolic regurgitant murmur is audible

along the LLSB. The systolic murmur of MR may be audible at the apex. A middiastolic rumble at the LLSB or at the apex (from relative stenosis of the tricuspid and/or mitral valve) and gallop rhythm may be present.

3. The ECG finding of left anterior hemiblock (or superior QRS axis) with the QRS axis between −40 degrees and −150 degrees is characteristic. RVH or RBBB is present in all, and many have LVH as well. Prolonged PR interval (first-degree AV block) is common.

4. CXR films always show cardiomegaly with increased PVMs.

5. 2D echo and color flow Doppler studies allow imaging of all components of ECD, as well as an assessment of the severity of the defect.

6. CHF occurs 1 to 2 months after birth, and recurrent pneumonia is commonly seen. Most patients without surgical intervention die in 2 to 3 years. The survivors develop PVOD and die in late childhood or as young adults.

Management

Medical: Medical management is recommended initially for small infants with CHF, as surgical mortality is relatively high in this age group. SBE prophylaxis is indicated.

Surgical

a. Palliative: PA banding may be carried out (but with a relatively high risk) in small infants if no significant MR is present.

b. Corrective: Closure of ASD and VSD and reconstruction of cleft AV valves under cardiopulmonary bypass and/or deep hypothermia carries surgical mortality of 5% to 10%. Timing varies with institutions and depends on the hemodynamic severity of the patients (ranging from a few months to several years of age). CHF unresponsive to aggressive medical therapy, repeated pneumonia with failure to thrive, and a large L-R shunt with pulmonary hypertension or increasing PVR are indications for surgery. Patients with Down syndrome develop PVOD early, requiring surgery earlier than those without Down syndrome.

Postsurgical: SBE prophylaxis is usually indicated even after surgery. Anticongestive medications and some restriction of activities may be required if residual hemodynamic abnormalities are present.

E. Partial Endocardial Cushion Defect (Ostium Primum ASD)

Prevalence: 1% to 2% of all CHD (much lower than secundum ASD).

Pathology and Pathophysiology: A defect is present in the lower part of the atrium septum near the AV valves. Clefts of the mitral and occasionally of the tricuspid valve are present. Pathophysiology is similar to that of ostium secundum ASD.

Clinical Manifestations

1. Usually asymptomatic during childhood.
2. Physical findings are identical to those of secundum ASD, except a regurgitant systolic murmur of MR, which may be present at the apex.
3. The ECG shows left anterior hemiblock, or superior QRS axis, as in complete ECD. First-degree AV block (50%) and RVH or RBBB (rsR′ pattern in V1) are common.
4. CXR findings are identical to those of secundum ASD except for the enlargement of the LA and LV when MR is significant.
5. 2D echo allows accurate diagnosis of primum ASD by direct imaging of the defect in the lower portion of the atrial septum.
6. CHF may develop in childhood and pulmonary hypertension in adulthood. Infective endocarditis, usually of AV valves, and arrhythmias (20%) may complicate the defect.

Management

Medical: No exercise restriction is required. SBE prophylaxis should be observed on indications.

Surgical: Closure of the ASD and reconstruction of the cleft mitral and tricuspid valves under cardiopulmonary bypass are performed electively at 1 to 2 years in children with no symptoms and earlier in infants with CHF or MR. Surgical mortality is approximately 3%.

Postsurgical: No restriction of activities. SBE prophylaxis is continued even after surgery. Sinus node dysfunction may develop and require pacemaker therapy.

F. Partial Anomalous Pulmonary Venous Return

Prevalence: Less than 1% of all children with CHD.

Pathology and Pathophysiology: One or more but not all PVs drain into the RA or its venous tributaries such as the SVC, IVC, coronary sinus, or left innominate vein. The hemodynamic alteration is similar to that in ASD.

Clinical Manifestations

1. Children with PAPVR are usually asymptomatic.
2. Physical findings are similar to those of ASD. When associated with ASD, the S2 is split widely and fixed. When the atrial septum is intact, the S2 is normal.
3. The ECG shows RVH or RBBB or is normal.
4. CXR films show RAE, RVE, and increased PVMs.
5. Echo diagnosis of PAPVR is less reliable.
6. If PAPVR is undetected, cyanosis and exertional dyspnea may develop during the third and fourth decades, resulting from pulmonary hypertension and PVOD.

Management

Medical: Exercise restriction is not required. SBE prophylaxis is probably not indicated.

Surgical: Surgical correction is carried out under cardiopulmonary bypass, usually when the patient is 2 to 5 years of age. A significant L-R shunt with Qp/Qs greater than 1.5:1 or 2:1 is an indication for surgery. Isolated single lobe anomaly is not ordinarily corrected.

Postsurgical: Restriction of activities is not indicated. SBE prophylaxis is not indicated beyond 6 months after surgery.

II. OBSTRUCTIVE LESIONS

A. Pulmonary Stenosis

Prevalence: 5% to 8% of children with CHDs.
Pathology and Pathophysiology

1. PS may be valvular (90%), subvalvular (infundibular), or supravalvular (i.e., stenosis of the PA). Dysplasia of the pulmonary valve is frequently seen with Noonan syndrome. Isolated infundibular PS is uncommon, usually associated with a large VSD (i.e., TOF).

2. A poststenotic dilatation of the MPA usually develops in valvular PS. Depending on the severity of PS, a varying degree of RVH develops. Dilatation of the RV does not result unless CHF supervenes.

Clinical Manifestations

1. Usually asymptomatic with mild PS. Exertional dyspnea and easy fatigability may be seen in moderately severe cases and CHF in severe cases. Newborns with critical PS are cyanotic and tachypneic.

2. An ejection click is present at the ULSB with valvular PS. The S2 may split widely, and the P2 may be diminished in intensity. A systolic ejection murmur (grade 2 to 5/6) with or without systolic thrill is best audible at the ULSB and transmits fairly well to the back and the sides. The louder and longer the murmur, the more severe is the stenosis. Neonates with critical PS may have only a faint heart murmur, if any.

3. The ECG is normal in mild PS. RAD and RVH are present in moderate PS. RAH and RVH with strain are present in severe PS. Neonates with critical PS may show LVH (due to hypoplastic RV and relatively large LV).

4. CXR findings: The heart size is usually normal, but the MPA segment may be prominent (i.e., poststenotic dilatation). PVMs are normal but may be decreased in severe PS.

5. 2D echo may show thick pulmonary valves with restricted systolic motion (doming) and a poststenotic dilatation of the MPA. The Doppler study can estimate the pressure gradient.

6. The severity of the obstruction tends to progress, especially with moderate or severe PS. CHF and sudden death are possible in patients with severe PS.

Management

Medical

a. Restriction of activity is usually not indicated except for severe PS.

b. SBE prophylaxis should be observed on indications.

c. Balloon valvuloplasty (performed at the time of cardiac catheterization) is the procedure of choice for significant pulmonary valve stenosis (when systolic pressure gradient is 50 mm Hg or greater). This procedure is useful even for dysplastic pulmonary valve.

d. For neonates with critical PS, prostaglandin E_1 (PGE,) infusion to reopen the ductus should be started and percutaneous balloon valvotomy may be performed; if it is not successful, surgery is indicated.

Surgical

a. In children with RV pressure greater than 80 mm Hg in whom balloon valvuloplasty is unsuccessful, pulmonary valvotomy is performed under cardiopulmonary bypass. Surgical mortality is less than 1%.

b. Patch widening of the RVOT and resection of the infundibular muscle may be indicated for infundibular PS. Dysplastic pulmonary valve often requires complete excision of the valve.

c. Neonates with critical PS may require a transventricular valvotomy while receiving PGE_1 infusion (with left Gore-Tex shunt if severe infundibular hypoplasia is present). Surgical mortality is about 10%.

Postsurgical: SBE prophylaxis should be observed on indications. Periodic echo studies are indicated to detect recurrences of the stenosis.

B. Aortic Stenosis

Prevalence: 5% of all CHD, with male preponderance (4:1).

Pathology and Pathophysiology

1. The stenosis may be at the valvular (most common), subvalvular, or supravalvular level. A bicuspid aortic valve is the most common form of AS. Supravalvular stenosis is often associated with William syndrome (mental retardation, characteristic "elfin facies," and PA stenosis). Subvalvular stenosis may be due to a simple diaphragm (discrete) or a long, tunnel-like narrowing of the LV outflow tract. Another type of subvalvular stenosis, IHSS, is a primary disorder of the heart muscle (cardiomyopathy).

2. Hypertrophy of the LV may develop if the stenosis is severe. A poststenotic dilatation of the ascending aorta develops with valvular AS. AR usually develops in subaortic AS.

Clinical Manifestations

1. Patients are asymptomatic with mild to moderate AS. Exertional chest pain or syncope may occur with severe AS. CHF develops within the first few months of life with critical AS.

2. A systolic thrill is present at the URSB, in the suprasternal notch, or over the carotid arteries. An ejection click may be audible with valvular AS. A rough or harsh systolic ejection murmur (grade 2 to 4/6) is best audible at the 2RICS or 3LICS, with good transmission to the neck and frequently to the apex. A high-pitched, early diastolic decrescendo murmur due to AR may be audible in patients with bicuspid aortic valve and those with discrete subvalvular stenosis. A narrow pulse pressure is present in severe AS. A higher systolic pressure in the right arm than in the left arm is found in supravalvular AS.

3. Newborn infants with critical AS may develop CHF. The heart murmur may be absent or faint, and the peripheral pulses are weak and thready. The heart murmur becomes louder when CHF improves.

4. The ECG is normal in mild cases. LVH with or without a strain pattern is seen in more severe cases.

5. CXR films are usually normal in children, but a dilated ascending aorta may be seen occasionally in valvular AS. No significant cardiomegaly de-

velops unless CHF supervenes or unless AR is substantial.
6. Echo studies are diagnostic. 2D echo may show the
anatomy of the aortic valve (bicuspid, tricuspid, or
unicuspid) and that of subvalvular and supravalvular
AS. The Doppler examination can estimate the
pressure gradient in various forms of AS.
7. CHF may develop during the newborn period or later
in life with severe AS. Chest pain, syncope, and even
sudden death (1% to 2%) may occur in children with
severe AS. A significant increase in the pressure gradient often occurs with growth.

Management

Medical

a. Exercise restriction against sustained strenuous activity is recommended in children with moderate
to severe AS. Maintenance of good oral hygiene
and SBE prophylaxis on indications are important.
b. In critically ill newborns and infants with CHF, anticongestive measures with fast-acting inotropic
agents and diuretics and oxygen administration,
with or without PGE_1 infusion, are indicated.
c. Balloon valvuloplasty may be performed at the
time of cardiac catheterization on selected patients. The results are not so promising as for PS.

Surgical

a. Closed aortic valvotomy using calibrated dilators or
balloon catheter without CPB may be performed
in sick infants.
b. Under cardiopulmonary bypass the following procedures may be performed depending on the
anatomy: (1) aortic valve commissurotomy, (2) replacement with an artificial valve using prosthetic,
porcine, or allograft valves, (3) replacement with
pulmonary valve autograft (Ross procedure, which
may be better than other artificial valves; see Fig
4-2), (4) valve replacement following aortic root
enlargement (Konno procedure) for severe annular or tunnel-like narrowing, (5) excision of the
membrane for discrete subvalvular AS, or (6) wid-

ening of the stenotic area using a diamond-shaped fabric patch for discrete supravalvular AS.

c. Infants with CHF from critical AS should be operated on an urgent basis (with a mortality rate as high as 40%). Children with peak systolic pressure gradient of 50 to 80 mm Hg may be operated on an elective basis. Surgery is indicated in children with symptoms (chest pain, syncope) with a strain pattern on the ECG or abnormal exercise test, even with a systolic pressure gradient slightly less than 50 mm Hg. An early elective operation may be considered for subvalvular AS with AR.

Postsurgical: Restriction from competitive sports is recommended in children with moderate residual AS and/or AR. SBE prophylaxis should be observed on indications. Recurrence of discrete subaortic AS is frequent following surgical resection of the membrane.

C. Coarctation of the Aorta

Prevalence: 8% to 10% of CHD with male preponderance (2:1).

Pathology and Pathophysiology

1. There is a narrowing of the aorta, most commonly in the upper thoracic aorta. Up to 85% of patients with COA have bicuspid aortic valve.

2. In *symptomatic infants* with COA, the descending aorta is supplied by RV via PDA during fetal life. Other cardiac defects, such as aortic hypoplasia, abnormal aortic valve, VSD, PDA, and mitral valve anomalies, are often present. Collateral circulation is poorly developed.

3. In *asymptomatic children* with COA the descending aorta is supplied by the LV via aortic isthmus during fetal life. Associated anomalies are uncommon, except for bicuspid aortic valve. Good collateral circulation usually develops.

4. In symptomatic infants RVH, rather than LVH, is usually present on the ECG. During fetal life the RV is the dominant ventricle that supplies blood to the de-

scending aorta and placenta through the ductus arteriosus. With the RV supplying the descending aorta, the RV ends up handling more blood than the LV. Therefore, there is a greater degree of RV dominance at birth, with resulting RVH on the ECG. This RVH is gradually replaced by LVH by the time the patient is 2 years of age.

1. Symptomatic Infants

Clinical Manifestations

1. Signs of CHF (poor feeding, dyspnea) and renal failure (oliguria, anuria) with general circulatory shock may develop in the first 2 to 6 weeks of life.
2. A loud gallop is usually present, but heart murmur may be absent in sick infants. Owing to CHF, weak and thready pulses are present throughout.
3. The ECG usually shows RVH or RBBB rather than LVH.
4. CXR films show a marked cardiomegaly and signs of pulmonary edema or pulmonary venous congestion.
5. 2D echo shows the site and extent of the COA and other associated defects. The Doppler examination reveals a disturbed flow distal to the COA and signs of delayed emptying in the proximal aorta.
6. In symptomatic infants with COA, early death from CHF and renal failure is possible.

Management

Medical: Intensive anticongestive measures should be given with fast-acting inotropic agents (catechols), diuretics, and oxygen before surgical treatment. PGE_1 infusion may be indicated to reopen the ductus. Balloon angioplasty is controversial.

Surgical

a. If CHF develops, the need for surgery is urgent. Surgical procedure of choice varies from institution to institution. Resection and end-to-end anastomosis (preferable when possible), subclavian flap aortoplasty, or patch angioplasty is performed (Fig 3-3).
b. If there is a large associated VSD, one of the follow-

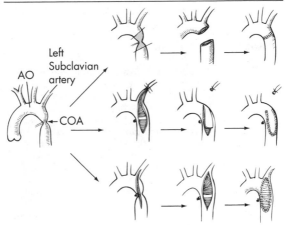

FIG. 3-3.
Surgical techniques for repair of COA. *Top,* End-to-end anastomosis. *Middle,* Subclavian flap procedure. *Bottom,* Patch aortoplasty. (From Park MK. *Pediatric Cardiology for Practitioners,* ed 3. St. Louis, Mosby, 1995.)

ing procedures may be performed. (1) COA repair without PA banding. If CHF persists, VSD closure is indicated. (2) PA banding at the time of COA repair. Later VSD repair and removal of the PA band when the patient is 6 to 24 months of age.

Postoperative

a. Reexamination every 6 to 12 months is indicated, since recoarctation is possible, especially if surgery is performed in the first year of life.

b. SBE prophylaxis should be continued on indications because of the frequently associated bicuspid aortic valve and residual coarctation.

c. Balloon angioplasty may be performed if a significant recoarctation develops.

d. Surveillance for and treatment of systemic hypertension are important.

2. Asymptomatic Children

Clinical Manifestations

1. These patients are usually asymptomatic except for occasional complaints of leg pain.
2. The pulse in the leg is absent or weak and delayed. Hypertension in the arm or higher BP readings in the arm than the thigh may be present. An ejection click resulting from bicuspid aortic valve is frequently audible at the apex and/or at the base. A systolic ejection murmur, grade 2 to 3/6, is audible at the URSB, MLSB, and in the left interscapular area in the back.
3. The ECG usually shows LVH, but it may be normal.
4. CXR films show normal or slightly enlarged heart. An E sign on the barium-filled esophagus or 3 sign on overpenetrated films may be found. Rib notching may be seen in children after about 5 years of age.
5. 2D echo may show a discrete shelflike membrane in the posterolateral aspect of the descending aorta. Bicuspid aortic valve is frequently imaged. The Doppler examination reveals disturbed flow and increased flow velocity distal to the coarctation.
6. Bicuspid aortic valve may cause stenosis and/or regurgitation later in life. If it is left untreated, LV failure, intracranial hemorrhage, or hypertensive encephalopathy may develop in childhood or adult life.

Management

Medical: Treatment of any hypertension is indicated. Balloon angioplasty of the COA may be performed, although it is controversial.

Surgical

a. Resection of the coarctation segment and end-to-end anastomosis constitute the procedure of choice. Other surgical options are illustrated in Figure 3-3.
b. COA with hypertension in the upper extremities or those with a prominent pressure gradient between

the arms and legs can be repaired electively when
the patient is 3 or 4 years old. Children with mild
COA (20 to 30 mm Hg) may be considered for surgery if a prominent pressure gradient develops
with exercise.

Postoperative

a. Annual examination with attention to (1) BP dif-
ferences in the arm and leg (recoarctation), (2)
persistence or resurgence of hypertension in the
arm *and* legs (cause not known), (3) associated abnormalities such as bicuspid aortic valve or mitral
valve disease, and (4) possible development of subaortic AS years after the surgery.

b. SBE prophylaxis should be observed on indications.

c. If COA recurs, balloon angioplasty may be performed.

D. Interrupted Aortic Arch

Prevalence: 1% of critically ill infants with CHDs.
Pathology and Pathophysiology

1. This extreme form of COA is divided into three types
according to the location of the interruption. In type
A (occurring in 30% of patients), the interruption
is distal to the left subclavian artery, type B (43%), between the left carotid and left subclavian arteries,
and type C (17%), between the innominate and left
carotid arteries.

2. PDA and VSD are almost always associated with this
defect. A bicuspid aortic valve (60%), mitral valve de-
formity (10%), persistent truncus arteriosus (10%),
or subaortic stenosis (20%) may be present.

Clinical Manifestations

1. Respiratory distress, cyanosis, poor peripheral pulse,
or circulatory shock develops in the first few days of
life.

2. Cardiac findings are nonspecific.

3. CXR films show cardiomegaly, increased PVMs, and
pulmonary edema. The upper mediastinum may be
narrow (due to the absence of thymus, i.e., DiGeorge
syndrome).

4. The ECG may show RVH.
5. Echo studies and angiocardiography are diagnostic.
   Management
1. Medical treatment consists of PGE_1 infusion, intubation, and oxygen administration. Work-up for DiGeorge syndrome (i.e., serum calcium) should be carried out.
2. Surgical repair of the interruption (primary anastomosis, vascular graft) and closure of a simple VSD are recommended if possible. If associated with complex defects, repair of the interruption and PA banding are performed with complete repair later.

III. CYANOTIC CONGENITAL HEART DEFECTS

A. Complete Transposition of the Great Arteries

Prevalence: TGA constitutes 5% of all CHD. It is more common in boys (3:1).

Pathology and Pathophysiology

1. The aorta (AO) arises anteriorly from the RV, and the PA arises posteriorly from the LV. The end result is complete separation of the two circuits, with hypoxemic blood circulating in the body and hyperoxemic blood circulating in the pulmonary circuit (Fig 3-4). Defects that permit mixing of the two circulations, such as ASD, VSD, and PDA, are necessary for survival. A VSD is present in 40% of cases. PS occurs in 30% to 35% of patients with VSD. The classic complete TGA is called D-transposition, in which the aorta is located anteriorly and to the right of the PA; hence, D-TGA. When the transposed aorta lies to the left of the PA, it is called L-transposition.
2. In neonates with poor mixing of the two circulations, progressive hypoxia and acidosis result in early death. CHF develops in the first week of life in many patients with this condition. The RV is the systemic ventricle, with resulting RVH on the ECG.

Clinical Manifestations

1. Cyanosis and signs of CHF (dyspnea, feeding difficulties) develop in the newborn period.

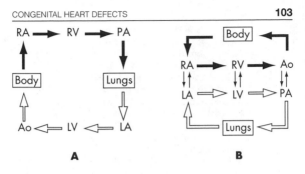

FIG. 3-4.
Circulation pathways of normal serial circulation **(A)** and parallel circulation of TGA **(B).** Open arrows indicate oxygenated blood, and solid arrows, desaturated blood.

2. Auscultatory findings are nonspecific. The S2 is single and loud. No heart murmur is audible in infants with an intact ventricular septum. When TGA is associated with VSD or PS, a systolic murmur of these defects may be audible.
3. Severe arterial hypoxemia unresponsive to oxygen inhalation and acidosis are present in infants with poor mixing. Hypoglycemia and hypocalcemia are occasionally present.
4. The ECG shows RAD and RVH. An upright T wave in V1 after 3 days of age may be the only abnormality suggestive of RVH. CVH may be present in infants with large VSD, PDA, or PS, as they produce an additional LVH.
5. CXR films show cardiomegaly with increased PVMs. An egg-shaped cardiac silhouette with a narrow superior mediastinum is characteristic.
6. 2D echo study is diagnostic. It fails to show a "circle-and-sausage" pattern of the normal great arteries in the parasternal short axis view. Instead, it shows two circular structures. Other views reveal the PA arising from the LV and the aorta arising from the RV. Associated anomalies (VSD, LVOT obstruction, PS, ASD, and PDA) are imaged.

7. Natural history and prognosis depend on anatomy.
   a. Infants with intact ventricular septum are the sickest group, but they demonstrate the most dramatic improvement following PGE_1 infusion or the Rashkind balloon atrial septostomy.
   b. Infants with VSD or large PDA are the least cyanotic group but are most likely to develop CHF and PVOD (as early as 3 or 4 months of age).
   c. Combination of VSD and PS allows considerably longer survival without surgery, but repair surgery carries a high risk.
   d. Cerebrovascular accident and progressive PVOD, particularly in infants with large VSD or PDA, are rare complications.

Management

Medical

   a. Metabolic acidosis, hypoglycemia, and hypocalcemia should be treated if present.
   b. PGE_1 infusion is started to raise arterial oxygen saturation by reopening the ductus.
   c. Administration of oxygen may help to raise systemic arterial oxygen saturation by lowering PVR and increasing PBF, with resulting increase in mixing.
   d. A therapeutic balloon atrial septostomy (Rashkind procedure) may be performed if immediate surgery is not planned.
   e. Treatment of CHF with digitalis and diuretics may be indicated.

   Surgical: Definitive surgeries consist of switching the right- and left-sided structures at the atrial level (Senning or Mustard operation), at the ventricular level (Rastelli operation), or at the great artery level (arterial switch operation).

   a. Intraatrial repair surgeries (e.g., Senning or Mustard operation) may result in obstruction to the pulmonary or systemic venous return (less than 5%), TR (rare), arrhythmias, and depressed RV function. Sudden death attributable to arrhythmias (3% of survivors) is a rare complication.

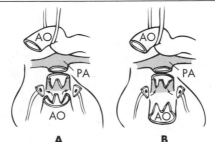

FIG. 3-5.
Arterial switch operation. **A,** The aorta is transected slightly above the coronary ostia, and the MPA is transected at about the same level. The ascending aorta is lifted, and both coronary arteries are removed from the aorta with triangular buttons **B,** Triangular buttons of similar size are made at the proper position in the PA trunk. **C,** The coronary arteries are transplanted to the PA. The ascending aorta is brought behind the PA and is connected to the the proximal PA to form a neoaorta. **D,** The triangular defects in the proximal aorta are repaired and the proximal aorta is connected to the PA. Note that the neopulmonary artery is in front of the neoaorta.

   b. Arterial switch, or the Jatene operation, is the procedure of choice in many cardiac centers (Fig 3-5).
Complications are much fewer with Jatene operation than with the intraatrial repair surgeries.

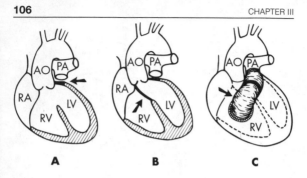

FIG. 3-6.
The Rastelli operation. **A,** The PA is divided from the LV, and the cardiac end is oversewn *(arrow)*. **B,** An intracardiac tunnel *(arrow)* is placed between the large VSD and the aorta. **C,** The RV is connected to the divided PA by an aortic homograft or a valve-bearing prosthetic conduit.

Possible complications include AR and late complication of coronary artery obstruction.
c. Rastelli operation (RV to PA connection) is indicated in patients with TGA + VSD + PS (Fig 3-6).
d. The Damus-Kaye-Stansel operation (Fig 3-7) is indicated for patients with TGA + VSD and subaortic stenosis.
e. The indication, timing, and type of surgical treatment vary greatly from institution to institution and are subject to change with the development of new information and new procedures. Fig 3-8 is a partial listing of many approaches used at this time.

Postsurgical
a. Patients who received the Senning or Mustard operation need to be followed closely for arrhythmias (quite common, more than 50%), sick sinus syndrome, TR, and depressed RV function.
b. Patients who received an arterial switch operation need to be followed for coronary artery ob-

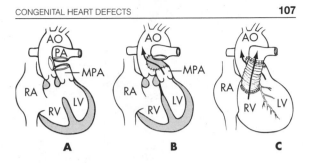

FIG. 3-7.
Damus-Kaye-Stansel operation for D-TGA + VSD + subaortic stenosis. **A,** D-TGA with VSD and subaortic stenosis. The MPA is transected near its bifurcation. An appropriately positioned and sized incision is made in the ascending aorta. **B,** The proximal MPA is anastomosed end to side to the ascending aorta, using either a Dacron tube or Gore-Tex. This channel will direct LV blood to the aorta. The aortic valve is either closed or left unclosed. **C,** Through a right ventriculotomy the VSD is closed, and a valved conduit is placed between the RV and the distal PA. This channel will carry RV blood to the PA.

       struction (with myocardial ischemia or infarction, LV dysfunction, and/or arrhythmias) and signs for AR.
   c. Limitation of activity may be indicated if arrhythmias or coronary insufficiency is present.
   d. SBE prophylaxis should be observed on indications.

B. Congenitally Corrected Transposition of the Great Arteries (L-TGA, Ventricular Inversion)

   Prevalence: Much less than 1% of all CHDs.
   Pathology and Pathophysiology
1. Visceroatrial relationship is normal (the RA on the right of the LA). The RA empties into the anatomic LV through the mitral valve, and the LA empties into the RV through the tricuspid valve. For this to occur

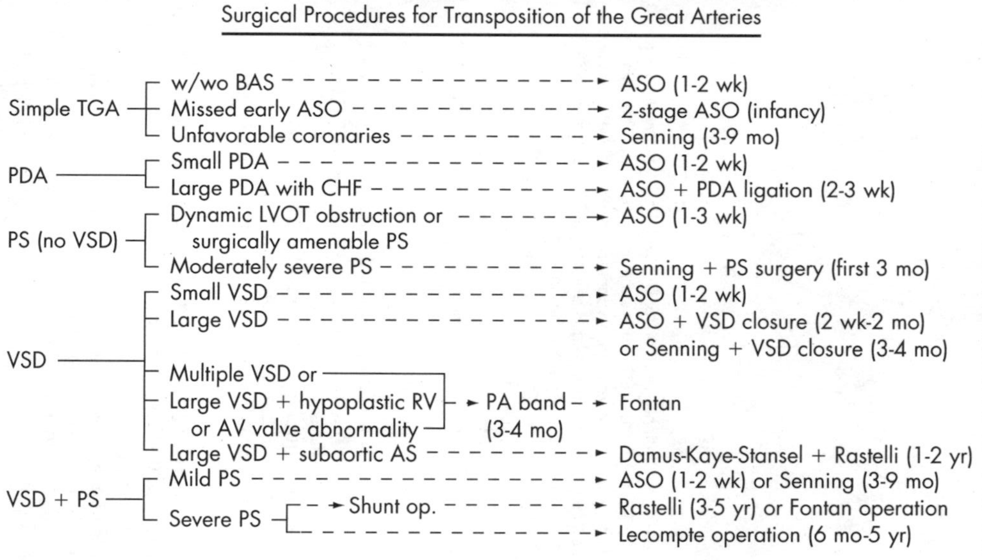

Surgical Procedures for Transposition of the Great Arteries

Simple TGA
- w/wo BAS → ASO (1-2 wk)
- Missed early ASO → 2-stage ASO (infancy)
- Unfavorable coronaries → Senning (3-9 mo)

PDA
- Small PDA → ASO (1-2 wk)
- Large PDA with CHF → ASO + PDA ligation (2-3 wk)

PS (no VSD)
- Dynamic LVOT obstruction or surgically amenable PS → ASO (1-3 wk)
- Moderately severe PS → Senning + PS surgery (first 3 mo)

VSD
- Small VSD → ASO (1-2 wk)
- Large VSD → ASO + VSD closure (2 wk-2 mo) or Senning + VSD closure (3-4 mo)
- Multiple VSD or → Fontan
- Large VSD + hypoplastic RV or AV valve abnormality → PA band (3-4 mo) → Fontan
- Large VSD + subaortic AS → Damus-Kaye-Stansel + Rastelli (1-2 yr)

VSD + PS
- Mild PS → ASO (1-2 wk) or Senning (3-9 mo)
- Severe PS → Shunt op. → Rastelli (3-5 yr) or Fontan operation
- → Lecompte operation (6 mo-5 yr)

FIG. 3-8.
Management flow diagram for TGA. ASO, arterial switch operation (Jatene operation); BAS, balloon atrial septostomy.

the LV lies to the right of the RV (i.e., ventricular inversion). The great arteries are transposed, with the aorta arising from the RV and the PA arising from the LV. The aorta lies to the left of and anterior to the PA (hence L-TGA). The final result is a functional correction: oxygenated blood coming into the LA goes to the anatomic RV and out the aorta.

2. Theoretically no functional abnormalities exist, but unfortunately most cases are complicated by associated defects, such as VSD (80%) with or without PS, resulting in cyanosis. Regurgitation of the systemic AV valve (tricuspid) occurs in 30% of the patients. Varying degrees of AV block, which are sometimes progressive, and SVT are also frequent.

Clinical Manifestations

1. Patients with associated defects are symptomatic during the first few months of life with cyanosis (VSD + PS) or CHF (large VSD). Patients without associated defects are asymptomatic.

2. The S2 is single and loud. A grade 2 to 4/6 harsh holosystolic murmur along the LLSB may indicate a VSD or the systemic AV valve (tricuspid) regurgitation. A grade 2 to 3/6 systolic ejection murmur at the ULSB or URSB may indicate PS.

3. Characteristic ECG findings are the absence of Q waves in V5 and V6 and/or the presence of Q waves in V4R or V1. Varying degrees of AV block, including complete heart block, may be present. Atrial and/or ventricular hypertrophy may be present in complicated cases.

4. CXR films may show characteristic straight left upper cardiac border (formed by the ascending aorta). Cardiomegaly and increased PVMs suggest associated VSD. Dextrocardia is frequent (50%).

5. 2D echo is diagnostic of the condition and associated defects.

6. Clinical course is determined by the presence or absence of associated defects and complications, some requiring surgeries. TR develops in about 30% of patients. Progressive AV conduction distur-

bances, including complete heart block (up to 30%), may occur.

Management

Medical

a. Treatment of any CHF and arrhythmias is indicated.

b. SBE prophylaxis should be used if indicated.

Surgical

a. Palliative procedures: PA banding for uncontrollable CHF due to a large VSD or an S-P shunt for patients with severe PS.

b. Corrective procedures include closure of VSD (with frequent complication of complete heart block), relief of PS, and/or valve replacement for significant TR.

c. Pacemaker implantation is indicated for complete heart block, either spontaneous or surgically induced.

Postsurgical: Regular follow-up is needed for a possible progression of AV block and for the routine pacemaker care if a pacemaker is implanted. Limitation of activity is indicated if hemodynamic abnormalities persist.

C. Tetralogy of Fallot

Prevalence: 10% of all CHD. It is the most common cyanotic CHD beyond infancy.

Pathology and Pathophysiology

1. The original description of TOF included four abnormalities: a large VSD, RVOT obstruction, RVH, and an overriding of the aorta. However, only two abnormalities are important: a VSD large enough to equalize pressures in both ventricles and an RVOT obstruction. The VSD is a perimembranous defect with extention into the infundibular septum. The RVOT may be in the form of infundibular stenosis (50%), pulmonary valve stenosis (10%), or both (30%). The pulmonary annulus and the PA are usually hypoplastic. In the most severe form of the

anomaly the pulmonary valve is atretic (10%). Right aortic arch is present in 25% of the cases.

2. Because of the nonrestrictive VSD, systolic pressures in the RV and the LV are identical. Depending on the degree of the RVOT obstruction, an L-R, bidirectional, or R-L shunt is present. With a mild PS, an L-R shunt is present (acyanotic TOF). With a more severe degree of PS, a predominant R-L shunt occurs (cyanotic TOF). The heart murmur audible in cyanotic TOF originates from the RVOT obstruction rather than the VSD.

Clinical Manifestations

1. Most patients are symptomatic, with cyanosis, clubbing, dyspnea on exertion, squatting, or hypoxic spells. Patients with acyanotic TOF may be asymptomatic.

2. A right ventricular tap and a systolic thrill at the lower and middle LSB are usually found. An ejection click of aortic origin, a loud and single S2, and a loud (grade 3 to 5/6) systolic ejection murmur at the middle and upper LSB are present. Occasionally a continuous murmur representing PDA shunt may be audible in a deeply cyanotic neonate who has TOF with pulmonary atresia. In the acyanotic form, a long systolic murmur resulting from VSD and infundibular stenosis is audible along the entire LSB and cyanosis is absent. (Thus, clinical findings of acyanotic TOF resemble those of a small-shunt VSD, but the ECG shows RVH or CVH).

3. The ECG shows RAD and RVH. CVH may be seen in the acyanotic form.

4. In cyanotic TOF, CXR films show normal heart size, decreased PVMs, and a boot-shaped heart with a concave MPA segment. Right aortic arch is present in 25% of the cases. CXRs of acyanotic TOF are indistinguishable from those of a small to moderate VSD.

5. 2D echo shows a large subaortic VSD and an overriding of the aorta. The anatomy of the RVOT, pulmonary valve, and pulmonary arteries can be imaged.

6. Children with the acyanotic form of TOF gradually develop the cyanotic form by 1 to 3 years of age. Hypoxic spells may develop in infants (see next section). Brain abscess, cerebrovascular accident, and SBE are rare complications. Polycythemia is common, but relative iron deficiency anemia (hypochromic) with normal hematocrit may be present. Coagulopathies are late complications of a longstanding severe cyanosis.

Hypoxic Spell

Hypoxic spell (also called cyanotic spell or "tet" spell) of TOF requires recognition and treatment, as it can lead to serious CNS complications. It occurs in young infants, with peak incidence between 2 and 4 months of age. It is characterized by (1) a paroxysm of hyperpnea (rapid and deep respiration), (2) irritability and prolonged crying, (3) increasing cyanosis, and (4) decreased intensity of the heart murmur. A severe spell may lead to limpness, convulsion, cerebrovascular accident, or even death.

Pathophysiology of Hypoxic Spell: In TOF, the RV and LV can be considered as a single pumping chamber, since there is a large VSD equalizing pressures in both ventricles. Lowering of the SVR or increasing resistance at the RVOT can increase the R-L shunting, and this in turn stimulates the respiratory center to produce hyperpnea. Hyperpnea results in an increase in systemic venous return, which in turn increases the R-L shunt through the VSD, as there is an obstruction at the RVOT. A vicious circle becomes established (Fig 3-9).

Treatment of the hypoxic spell is aimed at breaking the vicious circle. One or more of the following may be employed in decreasing order of preference:

1. Pick up and hold the infant over the shoulder or hold the infant in a knee-chest position.
2. Morphine sulfate 0.1 to 0.2 mg/kg SC or IM suppresses the respiratory center and abolishes hyper-

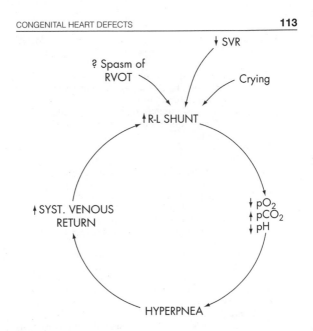

FIG. 3-9.
Mechanism of hypoxic spell. (From Park MK: *Pediatric Cardiology for Practitioners,* ed 3. St. Louis, Mosby, 1995.)

pnea. Do not try to establish an IV line initially; use the subcutaneous route for morphine.
3. Treat acidosis with sodium bicarbonate 1 mEq/kg IV. This reduces the respiratory center–stimulating effect of acidosis.
4. Oxygen inhalation has only limited value, since the problem is a reduced PBF, not the ability to oxygenate.

With these treatments the infant usually becomes less cyanotic and the heart murmur becomes louder, indicating improved PBF. If not fully responsive with the above measures:

5. Ketamine 1 to 3 mg/kg (average of 2 mg/kg) slow IV push works well (by increasing the SVR and sedating the infant).
6. Vasoconstrictors, such as phenylephrine (Neo-Synephrine) 0.02 mg/kg IV may work by raising the SVR and forcing more blood to the lungs.
7. Propranolol 0.01 to 0.25 mg/kg (average 0.05 mg/kg) slow IV push reduces the heart rate and may reverse the spell.

Management

Medical

a. Hypoxic spells should be recognized and appropriately treated.
b. Oral propranolol 2 to 4 mg/kg/day may be used to prevent hypoxic spells and to delay corrective surgery. The beneficial effect of propranolol may be related to its stabilizing action on peripheral vascular reactivity.
c. Maintenance of good oral hygiene and antibiotic prophylaxis against SBE are important.
d. Detection and treatment of relative iron deficiency anemia. Anemic children are particularly prone to CVA.

Surgical

a. Palliative procedures are indicated to increase PBF in infants with severe cyanosis or uncontrollable hypoxic spells, on whom the corrective surgery cannot safely be performed, and in children with hypoplastic PA, on whom the corrective surgery is technically difficult. Different types of S-P shunts have been performed (Fig 3-10).

   1) The Blalock-Taussig shunt (anastomosis between the subclavian artery and the ipsilateral PA) may be performed in older infants.
   2) Gore-Tex interposition shunt between the subclavian artery and the ipsilateral PA (modified Blalock-Taussig shunt) is the procedure of choice in small infants.
   3) Waterston shunt (anastomosis between the ascending aorta and the right PA) is no longer

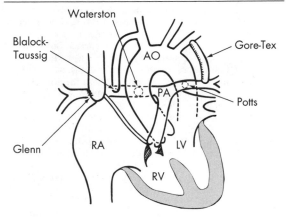

FIG. 3-10.
Palliative procedures for patients with cyanotic cardiac defects and decreased PBF. The Glenn procedure (anastomosis between the SVC and the right PA) may be performed in older infants with hypoplastic RV, as is seen with tricuspid atresia. (From Park MK: *Pediatric Cardiology for Practitioners,* ed 3. St. Louis, Mosby, 1995.)

        popular because of many complications following the operation.

    4) Potts operation (anastomosis between the descending aorta and the left PA) is rarely performed.

  b. Conventional repair surgery

    1) Symptomatic or cyanotic infants with favorable anatomy of the RVOT and PAs may have primary repair at any time after 3 to 4 months of age. Some centers perform primary repair even in younger infants, including newborns. Asymptomatic and minimally cyanotic children may have repair between ages 3 and 24 months, depending on the degree of the annular and

pulmonary hypoplasia. Mildly cyanotic infants
who have had previous shunt surgery may have
total repair at 1 to 2 years of age.

2) Total repair of the defect is carried out under
cardiopulmonary bypass. The procedure
includes patch closure of the VSD, widening of
the RVOT by resection of the infundibular
muscle tissue, and usually placement of a fabric
patch to widen the RVOT.

c. Rastelli operation is performed when there is severe hypoplasia or atresia of the RVOT. In this operation the VSD is closed with a patch and the RV
is connected to the PA by an aortic homograft or
a valve-bearing prosthetic conduit (Fig 3-6). This
procedure is performed when the patient is about
age 5, the mortality is 5% to 10%.

Postsurgical

a. Varying levels of activity limitation may be indicated.

b. SBE prophylaxis should be used if indicated on every patient who had TOF repair.

c. Arrhythmias, particularly ventricular tachycardia,
may develop later, and may be the cause of sudden
death. Holter monitoring, antiarrhythmic agents,
and pacemaker therapy may be indicated.

D. Tetralogy of Fallot with Pulmonary Atresia

Prevalence: About 10% of patients with TOF.
Pathology

1. In this extreme form of TOF, the intracardiac pathology resembles that of TOF in all respects except for
the presence of pulmonary atresia.

2. In two thirds of cases the PBF is mediated through the
PDA, which courses downward from the aortic arch
("vertical" ductus). In a third of cases the PBF is
through multiple systemic collaterals arising from the
aorta. Pulmonary arteries are hypoplastic and often
nonconfluent and have abnormal distribution (ar-
borization).

Clinical Manifestations

1. The patient is cyanotic at birth; the degree of cyanosis depends on whether the ductus is patent and how extensive the systemic collateral arteries are.
2. Usually no heart murmur is audible, but a faint, continuous murmur of PDA may be audible. The S2 is loud and single.
3. The ECG shows RAD and RVH.
4. CXR film shows normal heart size, often with a boot-shaped silhouette and a markedly decreased PVM ("black" lung field).
5. Echo studies are diagnostic of the condition, but angiocardiogram is necessary for complete delineation of the pulmonary artery anatomy and the collaterals.

Management

Medical

a. PGE₁ IV infusion is started to keep the ductus open for cardiac catherization and in preparation for surgery. The starting dose (Prostin VR pediatric solution) is 0.05 to 0.1 µg/kg/min. When the desired effect is obtained, the dosage is reduced step by step to 0.01 µg/kg/min.
b. Emergency cardiac catheterization is performed to delineate anatomy of the pulmonary arteries and systemic arterial collaterals.

Surgical

a. Primary surgical repair (closure of the VSD, conduit between the RV and the central PA) is possible only when a central PA of adequate size exists and the central PA connects without obstruction to sufficient regions of the lungs (at least equal to one whole lung). The overall hospital mortality varies between 5% and 20%.
b. Staged repair consists of the initial S-P shunts to induce the growth of the central PA before 1 or 2 years of age, followed by a surgical connection between or among the isolated regions of the lungs (termed unifocalization of pulmonary blood flow) before 3 or 4 years of age. The hospital mortality

of the unifocalization is 5% to 15%. Later, a conduit between the RV and a newly created central
pulmonary artery can be made. About a quarter to
half of the original patients can undergo the final
procedure.
  c. Occlusion of systemic collateral arteries is done by
     coil embolization preoperatively or at the time of
     surgery.
    Postsurgical: Frequent follow-up is needed to assess
       the palliative surgery, to decide appropriate time
       for further surgeries, and to determine an appro-
       priate time for conduit replacement. SBE prophy-
       laxis is indicated for an indefinite time. A certain
       level of activity restriction is needed for most pa-
       tients.

E. Tetralogy of Fallot with Absent Pulmonary Valve

  Prevalence: Approximately 2% to 6% of patients
    with TOF.
  Pathology and Pathophysiology
  1. The pulmonary valve leaflets are either absent or ru-
     dimentary, and the annulus is stenotic, usually associ-
     ated with TOF. A massive aneurysmal dilatation of
     the PAs results in fetal life, which compresses anteri-
     orly the lower end of the developing trachea and
     bronchi throughout the fetal life, producing signs of
     airway obstruction and respiratory difficulties in
     infancy. Pulmonary complications (e.g., atelectasis,
     pneumonia), rather than the intracardiac defect, are
     the usual cause of death. In some patients the duc-
     tus arteriosus is absent, with a more severe aneurys-
     mal dilation of the PAs.
  2. Since the annular stenosis is only moderate, an initial
     bidirectional shunt becomes predominantly an L-R
     shunt beyond the newborn period.
  Clinical Manifestations
  1. Mild cyanosis may be present in the newborn, but cy-
     anosis disappears and signs of CHF may develop when
     the PVR falls beyond the newborn period.
  2. A to-and-fro murmur ("sawing-wood sound") at the

upper and middle LSB (resulting from PS and PR) is characteristic of the condition. The S2 is loud and single, and RV hyperactivity is palpable.

3. The ECG shows RAD and RVH.

4. CXR films reveal a markedly dilated MPA and hilar PAs. The heart size is either normal or mildly enlarged, and PVMs may be slightly increased. The lung fields may show hyperinflated or atelectatic areas.

5. Echo confirms the diagnosis.

6. Most infants with severe pulmonary complications (e.g., atelectasis, pneumonia) die during infancy if treated only medically. The surgical mortality of infants with pulmonary complications is as high as 40%. Infants who survive infancy without serious pulmonary problems do well for 5 to 20 years, but they become symptomatic later and die of intractable right heart failure.

Management

> *Medical:* In the past medial management was preferred because of poor surgical results in the newborn period, but the mortality of medical management is very high. Once the pulmonary symptoms appear, neither surgical nor medical management carries good results.

> *Surgical:* Early surgical treatment (before respiratory symptoms develop) is advocated to reduce the effect of the compression by the PA aneuryms on the tracheobronchial trees.

a. Two-stage operation: Initially, ligation or tight banding of the MPA is performed to eliminate PR and excessive RV stroke output and to reduce further PA dilation, along with a Gore-Tex shunt. When the patient is age 2 to 4, closure of the VSD, reconstruction of the PA, and occlusion of the shunt are carried out. Some use a homograft valve at the pulmonary valve position, and others do not.

b. Primary repair: With recent advances in infant cardiac surgery, complete primary repair of the defect before respiratory symptoms develop may be the procedure of choice.

F. Total Anomalous Pulmonary Venous Return

Prevalence: 1% of all CHD. There is marked male preponderance (4:1) in the infracardiac type.

Pathology and Pathophysiology

1. The PVs drain into the RA or its venous tributaries rather than into the LA. The defects may be divided into the following four types (Fig 3-11).
   a. Supracardiac (50%): The common PV drains into the SVC via the left SVC (vertical vein) and the left innominate vein.
   b. Cardiac (20%): The common PV drains into the coronary sinus or the PVs enter the RA separately through four openings.
   c. Infracardiac (subdiaphragmatic) (20%): The common PV drains to the portal vein, ductus venosus, hepatic vein, or the IVC.
   d. Mixed type (10%): A combination of the other types.

   An interatrial communication (ASD or patent foramen ovale) is necessary for survival. The left side of the heart is relatively small.

2. Pulmonary venous return reaches the RA, in which systemic and pulmonary venous blood are completely mixed. Blood then goes to the LA through an ASD as well as to the RV. Thus, oxygen saturations in the systemic and pulmonary circulations are the same, resulting in systemic arterial desaturation. The level of systemic arterial oxygen saturation is proportional to the amount of PBF. When there is no obstruction to PV return (as seen in most of the supracardiac and cardiac types), PV return is large and the systemic arterial blood is only minimally desaturated. When there is obstruction to PV return, (as seen in the infracardiac type), PV return is small and the patient is extremely cyanotic, with signs of pulmonary edema on CXR films.

Clinical Manifestations without PV Obstruction

1. Growth retardation, mild cyanosis, history of pneumonia, and signs of CHF (tachypnea, tachycardia, hepatomegaly, and growth retardation) are common.

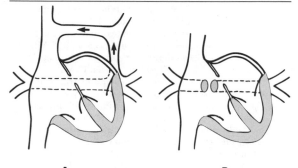

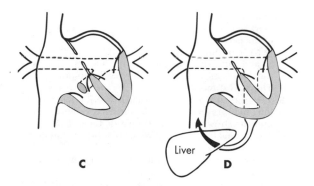

FIG. 3-11.

Anatomic classification of TAPVR. **A,** Supracardiac. **B,** Cardiac, draining into the RA. **C,** Cardiac, draining into the coronary sinus. **D,** Infracardiac.

2. Hyperactive RV impulse and characteristic quadruple or quintuple rhythm are present. The S2 is widely split and fixed and the P2 may be accentuated. A grade 2 to 3/6 systolic ejection murmur is usually

present at the ULSB. A middiastolic rumble is always present at the LLSB (from relative TS).

3. The ECG shows RAD, RVH (of "volume overload" type with rsR' pattern in V1), and occasional RAH.

4. CXR films show moderate to marked cardiomegaly (involving RA and RV) with increased PVMs. A "snowman" sign is seen in older infants (rarely before 4 months of age) with the supracardiac type.

5. 2D echo may demonstrate the common PV posterior to the LA without direct communication to the LA. A markedly dilated coronary sinus protruding into the LA (seen in TAPVR to the coronary sinus) or dilated left innominate vein and SVC (seen in the supracardiac type) may be imaged. An ASD and relatively small LA and LV are visualized.

6. CHF, growth retardation, and repeated pneumonias develop by 6 months of age.

Clinical Manifestations with PV Obstruction

1. Marked cyanosis and respiratory distress are present in the neonate.

2. Cardiac findings may be minimal. A loud and single S2 and gallop rhythm are present. Heart murmur is usually absent. Pulmonary rales may be audible.

3. The ECG shows RAD and RVH.

4. The heart size is usually normal on CXR films, but the lung fields reveal findings of pulmonary edema.

5. 2D echo shows relatively hypoplastic LA and LV. Anomalous PV return below the diaphragm can be directly visualized.

6. Patients with the infracardiac type rarely survive more than a few weeks without surgery.

Management for Patients Either with or without PV Obstruction

Medical

a. Intensive anticongestive measures with digitalis and diuretics are indicated for nonobstructive type.

b. Oxygen and diuretics are given for pulmonary edema in infants with obstructive type. Intubation and ventilator therapy with oxygen and positive end-expiratory pressure (PEEP) may be necessary in infants with severe pulmonary edema.

   c. Balloon atrial septostomy at the time of cardiac
      catheterization to enlarge the interatrial communi-
      cation may be beneficial at least temporarily.

   Surgical: There is no palliative procedure. Correc-
      tive surgery is indicated for all patients with this
      condition. Procedures vary with the site of the
      anomalous drainage. The goal is to channel PV
      blood to the LA. Newborns with PV obstruction are
      operated in the newborn period, and infants with-
      out PV obstruction are operated by 4 to 12 months
      of age.

   Postsurgical: Follow-up is needed for late develop-
      ment of obstruction to PV return (10%) or atrial
      arrhythmias, including sick sinus syndrome. SBE
      prophylaxis is usually not indicated unless an ob-
      struction is present.

G. Tricuspid Atresia

  Prevalence: 1% to 2% of all CHD in infancy.
  Pathology and Pathophysiology

1. The tricuspid valve is absent and the RV and PA are
hypoplastic, with decreased PBF. The great arteries
are transposed in 30% and normally related in 70% of
the cases. Associated defects such as ASD, VSD, or
PDA are necessary for survival. In the most common
type (50%), a small VSD and PS (with hypoplasia of
the PAs) are present and the great arteries are
normally related. In the second most common type
the great arteries are transposed and the pulmonary
valve is normal sized (20%) (Fig 3-12). COA or
interrupted aortic arch is frequently associated
anomaly, more commonly seen with TGA.

2. Systemic venous return is shunted from the RA to the
LA, with resulting dilation and hypertrophy of the
RA. The LA and LV are large because they handle
both systemic and pulmonary venous returns. The de-
gree of cyanosis is inversely related to the amount of
PBF.

  Clinical Manifestations

1. Severe cyanosis, poor feeding, and tachypnea are
usual.

NO TGA   D-TGA

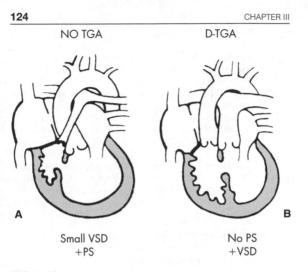

A   B

Small VSD   No PS
+PS   +VSD

FIG. 3-12.
Two most common types of tricuspid atresia. In about 50% of
patients, the great arteries are normally related and a small VSD and
PS are present **(A)**. When the great arteries are transposed (about
20% of all cases), a VSD is usually present without PS **(B)**.

2. The S2 is single. A grade 2 to 3/6 systolic regurgitant
   murmur of VSD is usually present at the LLSB. A continuous murmur of PDA is occasionally audible.
   Hepatomegaly is present when there is an inadequate
   interatrial communication or CHF.
3. The ECG shows characteristic "superior" QRS axis,
   RAH or CAH, and LVH.
4. CXR film shows normal or slightly increased heart
   size and decreased PVMs. A boot-shaped heart with
   concave MPA segment may be seen. In infants with
   TGA, PVMs may be increased.
5. 2D echo shows no functioning tricuspid valve, large
   LV, diminutive RV, and ASD. The presence or absence
   of TGA, VSD, PDA, and COA is also shown.

6. Few infants survive beyond 6 months of life without surgical palliation. Occasional patients with increased PBF develop CHF.

Management

Medical

a. PGE_1 IV infusion is indicated in severely cyanotic newborns to maintain the patency of the ductus.

b. The Rashkind procedure (balloon atrial septostomy) as a part of the initial cardiac catheterization may be performed to improve the R-L atrial shunt.

c. Infants with adequate size of VSD and normal PBF need to be followed closely for decreasing oxygen saturation resulting from reduction of the VSD.

Surgical

a. Most patients with tricuspid atresia require a palliative procedure to survive. The objective is to increase PBF in the newborn (by an S-P shunt operation) when it is deficient, and to diminish PBF (by PA banding) when it is excessive. In older infants, a "bidirectional" Glenn operation may be performed (Fig 3-13, *A*). In infants with TGA and a restrictive VSD, the Damus-Kaye-Stansel procedure (Fig 3-6) plus an S-P shunt may be preferred to the PA banding, which carried a high mortality.

b. A Fontan-type operation (Fig 3-13, *B*) is considered the definitive surgery. The cavocaval baffle-to-PA anastomosis with or without fenestration is the procedure of choice. Infants 4 years of age or older with normal PVR and PA pressure (mean pressure below 15 mm Hg), adequate PA size and normal LV function (ejection fraction above 60%) are considered good candidates for the Fontan-type operation, although it can be performed in younger children. Contraindications for the procedure include small or stenotic pulmonary arteries and an elevated PVR. Low cardiac output and/or heart failure are early postoperative complications. Persistent pleural effusion is also common.

Postsurgical: Long-term follow-up is needed for supraventricular arrhythmias, prolonged hepatomeg-

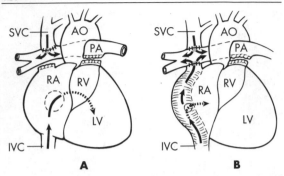

FIG. 3-13.
Bidirectional Glenn operation or SVC-RPA anastomosis **(A)** and cavocaval baffle-to-PA connection with or without fenestration **(B).**

aly, protein-losing enteropathy, and stenosis of the anastomosis sites. The patients should be on a low-salt diet, be excluded from competitive sports, and receive SBE prophylaxis on indications.

H. Pulmonary Atresia

Prevalence: Less than 1% of all CHDs
Pathology and Pathophysiology
1. The pulmonary valve is atretic and the interventricular septum is intact. An interatrial communication (either ASD or PFO) and PDA are necessary for survival.
2. The RV size is variable and is related to survival. In the *tripartite type,* all three (inlet, trabecular, and infundibular) portions of the RV are present and the RV is nearly normal in size. In the *bipartite type,* the inlet and infundibular portions are present (but the trabecular portion is obliterated). In the *monopartite type,* only the inlet portion is present. In the monopartite type, the RV is diminutive and coronary sinusoids are almost always present.

3. The high pressure in the RV is decompressed through dilated coronary sinusoids into the left or right coronary artery. TR is commonly present. The prevalence of the sinusoids is directly related to the RV pressure and inversely related to the amount of TR. The obstruction of the proximal coronary arteries, which is often present, may cause high surgical mortality.

4. Pathophysiology is similar to that of tricuspid atresia. The RA hypertrophies and enlarges to shunt systemic venous return to the LA. The LA and LV handle both systemic and pulmonary venous returns and therefore enlarge. PBF depends on the patency of PDA; closure of PDA after birth results in death.

Clinical Manifestations

1. Severe and progressive cyanosis is present from birth.

2. The S2 is single. Usually no heart murmur is present. A soft, continuous murmur of PDA may be audible at the ULSB.

3. The ECG shows normal QRS axis (in contrast to the "superior" QRS axis seen in tricuspid atresia), RAH, and LVH (monopartite type) or occasional RVH (tripartite type).

4. The heart size on CXR film may be normal or large (with RA enlargement). The MPA segment is concave, with markedly decreased PVMs.

5. 2D echo usually demonstrates the atretic pulmonary valve and hypoplasia of the RV cavity and tricuspid valve. The atrial communication and PDA can be imaged and their size estimated.

6. Prognosis is exceedingly poor without PGE_1 infusion and surgery.

Management

Medical

a. As soon as the diagnosis is suspected, PGE_1 IV infusion is started to maintain ductal patency.

b. Cardiac catheterization and angiocardiography are recommended for most patients to demonstrate coronary sinusoids (by RV angio) and to demonstrate possible coronary artery anomalies (by aortogram). A balloon atrial septostomy may be indicated to improve the R-L atrial shunt, but only in patients with RV sinusoids. The balloon atrial septostomy is not performed in patients with the tripartite type. Such patients may become candidates for RVOT patch, in which an elevated RA pressure is important to maximize RV forward output.

Surgical

a. Urgent initial procedures

There are three categories of surgical decision for this condition, depending on the RV size and the presence or absence of RV sinosoids or coronary artery anomalies.

1) When the RV appears adequate in size for future growth, a connection is established between the RV and the MPA, (either by transannular patch or closed transpulmonary valvotomy) in preparation for a two-ventricular repair. An S-P shunt is performed at the same time.

2) In patients with monopartite RV and sinusoids, an S-P shunt without the RV outflow patch is recommended because decompression of the RV (by valvotomy or an outflow patch) may reverse coronary flow into the RV, producing myocardial ischemia. Fontan operation can be performed later.

3) If coronary anomalies are identified by an aortogram, the sinusoids are left alone. If no coronary artery anomalies are identified, either sinusoidal ligation or closure of the tricuspid valve (thromboexclusion of the RV) may be performed. This increases the suitability for an eventual Fontan operation.

b. Follow-up procedures

1) For those who received the RVOT patch and an S-P shunt and who show evidence of growth of the RV cavity, the S-P shunt is closed if the patient tolerates balloon occlusion of the shunt during cardiac catheterization.

2) For those who received a closed pulmonary valvotomy and an S-P shunt and who have a large
   enough RV, an RVOT reconstruction and
   closure of ASD and the shunt are carried out.
3) For those who continue to have hypoplasia of
   the RV and tricuspid valve annulus, a Fontan-
   type operation is performed later.
4) An additional shunt operation may be necessary
   in patients on whom none of the above procedures can be performed.

Postsurgical: Most patients require close follow-up
because none of the surgical procedures are cura-
tive. SBE prophylaxis is used if indicated.

I. Ebstein Anomaly

Prevalence: Less than 1% of all CHDs.

Pathology and Pathophysiology

1. The septal and posterior leaflets of the tricuspid valve
   are displaced into the RV cavity, so that a portion of
   the RV is incorporated into the RA (atrialized RV), resulting in functional hypoplasia of the RV and TR
   (Fig 3-14). An interatrial communication is present,
   with resulting R-L atrial shunt.
2. The RA is massively dilated and hypertrophied. In addition, WPW syndrome is frequently associated with
   the anomaly and predisposes to attacks of SVT.

Clinical Manifestations

1. In severe cases cyanosis and CHF develop in the first
   few days of life, with some subsequent improvement.
   In milder cases dyspnea, fatigue, and cyanosis on
   exertion may be present in childhood.
2. The S2 is widely split. Characteristic triple or quadruple rhythm, consisting of split S1, split S2, S3, or S4, is
   present. A soft regurgitant systolic murmur of TR is
   usually audible at the LLSB.
3. Characteristic ECG findings are RBBB and RAH.
   WPW syndrome, SVT, and first-degree AV block are
   occasionally present.
4. CXR film shows extreme cardiomegaly, involving principally the RA, and decreased PVMs.

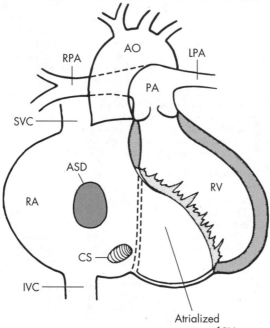

FIG. 3-14.
Ebstein anomaly of the tricuspid valve. There is a downward displacement of the tricuspid valve into the RV. Part of the RV is incorporated into the RA (atrialized portion of the RV). Regurgitation of the tricuspid valve results in an enlargement of the RA. An atrial septal defect is usually present.

5. 2D echo shows the apical displacement of the septal leaflet of the tricuspid valve. TR, a small RV cavity and a large RA, and an ASD are also imaged.

6. Cyanosis of newborns tends to improve as the PVR falls. Attacks of SVT are common. Other possible complications include CHF, LV dysfunction with fibrosis, brain abscess, cerebrovascular accident, and infective endocarditis.

Management

Medical

a. Administration of PGE_1 infusion and inotropic agents and correction of metabolic acidosis may be necessary in severely cyanotic newborns with the defect.

b. Anticongestive measures with digitalis and diuretics are indicated if CHF develops.

c. Treatment of SVT with digoxin alone or in combination with propranolol or other antiarrhythmic agents may be given.

Surgical: There is controversy concerning the surgical procedure.

a. Tricuspid annuloplasty (e.g., Danielson or Carpentier technique) is most desirable, although frequently limited by anatomy.

b. Tricuspid valve replacement with a prosthetic or tissue valve and closure of ASD is less desirable, but may be performed in patients who cannot have the annuloplasty.

c. A Fontan-type operation is advocated in patients with severely hypoplastic RV.

d. The Starnes operation may be performed in a critically ill newborn. In this operation the tricuspid valve is closed with the pericardium, the ASD is enlarged, and an S-P shunt is created. This is later followed by a Fontan-type operation.

e. For patients with WPW syndrome and recurrent SVT, surgical interruption of the accessory pathway is recommended at the time of surgery.

Postsurgical: Arrhythmias may persist even after surgery (in 10% to 20% of patients) requiring follow-up. SBE prophylaxis is recommended if indicated. Limitation of activities from competitive or strenuous sports may be indicated.

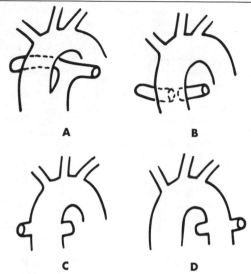

FIG. 3-15.
Anatomic types of persistent truncus arteriosus. **A,** type I. **B,** type II.
C, type III. **D,** type IV, or pseudotruncus arteriosus.

J. Persistent Truncus Arteriosus

Prevalence: Persistent truncus arteriosus constitutes
fewer than 1% of all CHDs.

Pathology and Pathophysiology

1. Only a single arterial trunk (with a truncal valve)
   leaves the heart and gives rise to the pulmonary,
   systemic, and coronary circulations. A large VSD is always present. A right aortic arch is present in 30%
   of patients. Anatomically, this anomaly is divided into
   four types (Fig 3-15): type I (affects 60%); type II,
   (20%); type III, (10%); and type IV, (10%). Coronary
   artery abnormalities (stenotic coronary ostia, abnor-

mal branching and course) are quite common, contributing to a high surgical mortality. DiGeorge syndrome with hypocalcemia is present in about 30% of patients.

2. The magnitude of PBF is usually increased in type I, normal in types II and III, and decreased in type IV. As is with other cyanotic CHDs, the level of systemic arterial oxygen saturation is directly related to the amount of PBF. Therefore, with decreased PBF cyanosis is notable. With increased PBF, cyanosis is minimal, but CHF may develop.

Clinical Manifestations

1. Cyanosis may be noted immediately after birth. Signs of CHF may develop within several weeks.

2. A grade 2 to 4/6 regurgitant systolic murmur (suggestive of VSD) is present along the LSB. A high-pitched diastolic decrescendo murmur of truncal valve regurgitation is occasionally present. An apical diastolic rumble with or without gallop rhythm may be audible when PBF is large. Wide pulse pressure and bounding arterial pulses may be present.

3. The ECG shows CVH (70% of patients); RVH or LVH is less common.

4. CXR films usually show cardiomegaly (biventricular and LA enlargement) and increased PVMs. A right aortic arch is seen in 30% of patients.

5. 2D echo demonstrates a large VSD directly under the truncal valve, similar to TOF. The pulmonary valve cannot be shown. A large single great artery arising from the heart (truncus) and the posterior branching of the PA from the truncus may be seen.

6. Without surgery, most infants die of CHF within 6 to 12 months. Clinical improvement occurs if the infant develops PVOD. Truncal valve regurgitation, if present, worsens with time.

Management

Medical: Vigorous anticongestive measures with digitalis and diuretics are required.

Surgical

a. PA banding may be indicated in small infants with

large PBF and CHF, but the mortality is high and the result not satisfactory. Primary repair of the defect may be preferable.

b. Rastelli procedure may be performed for type I during infancy (Fig 3-6). The VSD is closed so that the LV ejects into the truncus, and a valved conduit is placed between the RV and the PA. In Barbero-Marcial operation autologous tissue is used to correct type I truncus.

c. For types II and III the cuff of the truncal tissue including the PA orifices is excised. This cuff is connected to the distal end of a valved conduit.

d. Truncal valve replacement may be necessary for severe truncal regurgitation.

Postsurgical: Regular follow-up is needed for truncal valve regurgitation, adequacy of conduit and possible ventricular arrhythmias. SBE prophylaxis and limitation of activities from competitive sports are indicated.

K. Single Ventricle

Prevalence: Single ventricle constitutes fewer than 1% of all CHDs.

Pathology and Pathophysiology

1. Both AV valves empty into a common main ventricular chamber (double-inlet ventricle). A rudimentary infundibular chamber communicates with the main chamber through the bulboventricular foramen. One great artery arises from the main chamber, and the other usually arises from the rudimentary chamber. If the main chamber has anatomic characteristics of the LV (80%), it is called double-inlet LV. If the main chamber has anatomic characteristics of the RV, it is called double-inlet RV. Rarely both atria empty via a common AV valve into the main chamber (common-inlet ventricle). Either D- or L-TGA is present in 85% of patients, and AS or PS is common. The most common form of single ventricle is double-inlet LV with L-TGA in which the aorta arises from the rudimentary chamber (Fig 3-16). The bul-

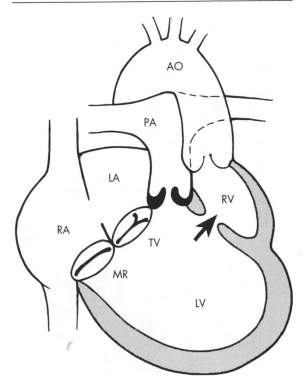

FIG. 3-16.
The most common form of single ventricle. The single ventricle is anatomic LV. The great arteries are transposed, with the aorta anterior to and left of the PA and the aorta arising from the rudimentary RV. Stenosis of the pulmonary valve is present in about 50% of patients (shown as thick valves). This type accounts for 70% to 75% of cases of single ventricle.

boventricular foramen is frequently obstructive, which has important hemodynamic and surgical implications (see Surgical Management). A high prevalence of asplenia or polysplenia syndrome is found.

2. There is a complete mixing of systemic and pulmonary venous blood in the ventricle, and therefore the oxygen saturation in the aorta and PA is identical. The systemic oxygen saturation is proportional to the amount of PBF. With decreased PBF (seen in patients with associated PS), marked cyanosis results. In patients without PS, PBF is large and the patient is minimally cyanotic and may develop CHF.

Clinical Manifestations

1. Cyanosis of a varying degree is present from birth. Symptoms and signs of CHF, failure to thrive, and bouts of pneumonia are commonly reported.

2. Physical findings depend on the magnitude of PBF. With increased PBF physical findings resemble those of TGA and VSD or even large VSD. With decreased PBF, physical findings resemble those of TOF.

3. ECG
   a. An unusual ventricular hypertrophy pattern with similar QRS complexes across most or all precordial leads (RS, rS, or QR pattern) appears.
   b. Abnormalities in the Q wave (due to abnormalities in septal depolarization) are also common. They take one of the following forms: (1) Q waves in the RPLs, (2) no Q waves in any precordial leads, or (3) Q waves in both the RPLs and LPLs.
   c. First- or second-degree AV block or arrhythmias may be present.

4. When PBF is increased, CXR film shows cardiomegaly and increased PVMs. When PBF is normal or decreased, the heart size is normal and the PVMs are normal or decreased.

5. 2D echo shows two distinct AV valves emptying into a single ventricular chamber. The rudimentary chamber is usually to the left of and anterior to the main chamber. Other anomalies described under pathology

are also imaged. The bulboventricular foramen is often obstructive (with pressure gradient above 10 mm Hg).

6. CHF with growth failure manifests in early infancy. Clinical improvement occurs if PVOD develops. Some infants develop obstruction of the foramen, with resulting deterioration in hemodynamics. These consist of increased PBF, decreased systemic perfusion, and hypertrophy of the main chamber with decreased compliance.

Management

Medical

a. Anticongestive measures with digitalis and diuretics are indicated.

b. Infants with severe PS or pulmonary atresia and those with interrupted aortic arch require PGE$_1$ infusion.

Surgical

a. An S-P shunt (for infants) or Glenn procedure (for children older than 2 years) may be required for patients with PS and severe cyanosis.

b. PA banding is performed in patients (without PS) and uncontrollable CHF if the foramen is not obstructive, but the patient should be watched closely for the development of obstruction of the foramen after the banding. If the foramen is obstructive, the patient does not tolerate the banding well (surgical mortality runs 25% to 50%).

c. If the foramen is small, one of the following two alternative porcedures can be performed: (1) Damus-Kaye anastomosis (transection of the MPA and anastomosis of the proximal PA to the aorta, and an S-P shunt or a cavopulmonary shunt) or (2) enlargement of the bulboventricular foramen.

d. A modified Fontan procedure may be performed when the patient is age 3 or 4 following closure of the tricuspid valve. The mortality is relatively high (20%-30%).

e. Attempts at septating the single ventricle are usually unsuccessful.

L. Double-Outlet Right Ventricle (DORV)

Prevalence: Less than 1% of all CHDs.

Pathology and Pathophysiology

1. The aorta and the PA arise side by side from the RV.
   The only outlet from the LV is a large VSD. The aortic and pulmonary valves are at the same level.
   Subaortic and subpulmonary conuses separate the
   aortic and pulmonary valves from the tricuspid and
   mitral valves, respectively. DORV may be subdivided
   according to the position of the VSD and further
   by the presence of PS.
   a. Subaortic VSD (50% to 70% prevalence). PS is
      common (50% prevalence) in this (Fallot) type.
   b. Subpulmonary VSD (Taussig-Bing anomaly).
   c. Doubly committed VSD.
   d. Remote VSD.
2. Pathophysiology of DORV is determined primarily by
   the position of the VSD and the presence or absence
   of PS.
   a. With subaortic VSD (Fig 3-17, *A*), oxygenated
      blood (open arrow) from the LV is directed to the
      aorta (AO) and desaturated systemic venous blood
      (solid arrow) is directed to the pulmonary artery
      (PA), producing mild or no cyanosis. The PBF is in-
      creased in the absence of PS resulting in CHF.
      Therefore, clinical pictures of this type resemble
      those of a large VSD with pulmonary hypertension
      and CHF.
   b. With subpulmonary VSD (Fig 3-17, *B*), oxygenated
      blood from the LV is directed to the PA, and de-
      saturated blood from the systemic vein is directed
      to the aorta, producing severe cyanosis. The PBF
      increases with the fall of the PVR. Clinical pictures
      therefore resemble those of TGA. PVOD devel-
      ops relatively early.
   c. In the presence of PS (Fallot type), clinical pictures
      resemble those of TOF (Fig 3-17, *C*).
   d. With the VSD close to both semilunar valves (dou-
      bly committed VSD) or remotely located from

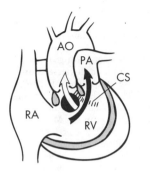
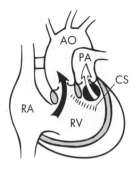

A

B

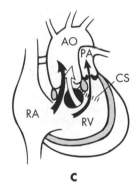

C

FIG. 3-17.

Three representative types of DORV, viewed with the RV free wall removed. **A,** Subaortic VSD. **B,** Subpulmonary VSD (Taussig-Bing anomaly). **C,** Subaortic VSD with PS. Doubly committed and remote VSDs are not shown. *AO,* aorta; *CS,* crista supraventricularis.

these valves (remote VSD), cyanosis of a mild degree is present and the PBF is increased.

Clinical Manifestations: Clinical manifestations vary greatly with the location of the VSD and the presence or absence of PS.

1. Subaortic VSD without PS: Physical findings resemble those of a large VSD with pulmonary hypertension and CHF. The ECG often resembles that of ECD ("superior" QRS axis, LAH, RVH, or CHF and occasional first-degree AV block). CXR films show cardiomegaly with increased PVMs and a prominent MPA segment.

2. Subpulmonary VSD (Taussig-Bing malformation): Physical findings resemble those of TGA with severe cyanosis in newborn infants. The ECG shows RAD, RAH, and RVH. LVH may be seen during infancy. First-degree AV block is frequently present. CXR films show cardiomegaly with increased PVMs.

3. Fallot-type DORV (with PS): Physical findings are similar to those seen in cyanotic TOF. The ECG shows RAD, RAH, and RVH or RBBB. CXR films show normal heart size (with upturned apex) and decreased PVMs.

4. Echo (for all types): Diagnostic 2D echo signs include: 1) both great arteries arising from the RV and running a parallel course in their origin, 2) absence of the LVOT and demonstration of a VSD, and 3) the mitral-semilunar discontinuity.

Management

Medical: Medical treatment of CHF and SBE prophylaxis if indicated.

Surgical

a. Palliative procedures

1) For infants with large PBF and CHF (e.g., remove VSD), a PA banding may be performed; for subaortic and doubly committed VSD, primary repair is a better choice.

2) For infants with subpulmonary VSD, enlarging the ASD by the balloon or blade atrial septectomy is important for better mixing of

pulmonary and systemic venous blood and decompression of the LA.

3) For infants with PS and decreased PBF (Fallot type), an S-P shunt is indicated.

b. Corrective surgeries

1) Subaortic VSD and doubly committed VSD: Creation of an intraventricular tunnel between the VSD and the subaortic outflow tract by 6 months of age without PA banding. The surgical mortality rate is 5% to 10%.

2) Subpulmonary VSD: An intraventricular tunnel between the subpulmonary VSD and the aorta is most desirable if technically feasible (mortality 15%). If that is not possible, an intraventricular tunnel between the VSD and the PA (turning it into TGA), plus the arterial switch (the Jatene) operation during the first month of life (surgical mortality 10% to 15%) or the Senning operation (surgical mortality above 40%).

3) Fallot type: An intraventricular tunnel procedure (VSD to aorta) plus relief of PS by a patch graft at 6 months to 2 years of age or a homograft valved conduit between the RV and the PA at 4 to 5 years of age.

4) Remote VSD: When possible, an intraventricular tunnel procedure (VSD to aorta) is preferred (mortality 30% to 40%). If that is not possible, either a Fontan-type operation (mortality 5%) or the Senning operation plus closure of the VSD plus LV-to-aorta valved conduit placement (surgical mortality about 15%) is performed.

M. Splenic Syndromes (Atrial Isomerism) (Asplenia Syndrome and Polysplenia Syndrome)

Prevalence: 1% of newborns with symptomatic CHD.

Pathology and Pathophysiology: There is a failure of differentiation into the right- and left-sided organs in splenic syndromes, with resulting congenital malformations of multiple organ systems. *Asplenia syndrome* (right atrial isomerism, Ivemark syndrome) is associated with the absence of the spleen, a left-sided organ, and a tendency to bilateral right-sidedness. In *polysplenia syndrome* (left atrial isomerism), multiple splenic tissues with a tendency for bilateral left-sidedness are present. Although the type and severity of cardiovascular malformations are somewhat different between the two syndromes, the same types of defects may be present in both conditions.

1. Noncardiac malformations
   a. In asplenia syndrome, bilateral three-lobed right lungs with bilateral eparterial bronchi and various gastrointestinal malformations, including a symmetric midline liver and malrotation of the intestines, are present. The stomach may be on the right or the left.
   b. In polysplenia syndrome, bilateral, bilobed lungs (two left lungs); bilateral, hyparterial bronchi; symmetric liver (25%); occasional absence of gallbladder; and some degree of intestinal malrotation (80%) are present.
2. Complex cardiac malformations are always present. Cardiovascular malformations involve all parts of the heart: systemic and pulmonary veins, the atria, the AV valves, the ventricles, and the great arteries. In general, asplenia syndrome has more severe abnormalities of these structures. A normal heart or only minimal malformation of the heart is present in up to 25% of the patients with polysplenia syndrome. Bilateral SVCs are common, and anomalies of the pulmonary venous return are usually present. Single atrium, secundum ASD, and primum ASD are all common. There are either two sinus nodes (asplenia) or no sinus node (polysplenia). The coronary sinus is usually absent. Single AV valve is common, especially in asplenia. Either a single ventricle or VSD is usually present. TGA is usually present in asplenia syndrome and occasionally in polysplenia syndrome.

   Cardiovascular anomalies that help to distinguish these two syndromes are summarized in Table 3-1.

TABLE 3-1.

Cardiovascular Malformations in Asplenia and Polysplenia Syndromes

Structure	Asplenia Syndrome	Polysplenia Syndrome
Systemic veins	Normal IVC in all but may be left-sided (35%) (azygos continuation almost never seen)	*Absent hepatic segment of IVC with azygos continuation, right or left (85%)
Pulmonary veins	*TAPVR with extracardiac connection (75%), often with PV obstruction	Normal PV return (50%) Right PVs to right-sided atrium; left PVs to left-sided atrium (50%)
Atrium and atrial septum	Bilateral right atria (bilateral sinus node) Primum ASD (100%) + secundum ASD (66%)	Bilateral left atria Single atrium, primum ASD (60%), or secundum ASD (25%)
AV valve	*Single AV valve (90%)	Normal AV valve (50%); single AV valve (15%)
Ventricles	Single ventricle (50%); two ventricles (50%)	*Two ventricles almost always present; VSD (65%); DORV (20%)
Great arteries	*Transposition (70%) (D-TGA, L-TGA)	Normal great arteries (85%); transposition (15%)
ECG	Stenosis (40%) or atresia (40%) of pulmonary valve Normal P axis, or in the +90 to +180° quadrant	Normal pulmonary valve (60%); pulmonary stenosis or atresia (40%) *Superior P axis (70%)

*Important differentiating points.

3. There is usually a complete mixing of systemic and pulmonary venous blood in the heart because of multiple cardiovascular malformations. When PBF is reduced, as in asplenia, severe cyanosis results. When PBF is increased, as in polysplenia syndrome, cyanosis is not intense and CHF often develops.

Clinical Manifestations

1. With asplenia syndrome cyanosis is often severe shortly after birth. Signs of CHF may develop during the neonatal period in polysplenia syndrome. Auscultation of the heart is nonspecific, but heart murmurs of VSD and/or PS are frequently audible. A symmetric liver (midline liver) is characteristic.

2. The ECG shows a "superior" QRS axis (due to ECD) in both conditions. An additional "superior" P axis (−30 to −90 degrees) strongly suggests polysplenia syndrome. In asplenia syndrome, the P axis may be either normal or alternating between the left lower and right lower quadrants (because two sinus nodes alternate the pacemaker function). RVH, LVH, or CVH is usually present. Complete heart block occurs in about 10% of the patients with polysplenia syndrome.

3. The heart size is normal or only slightly increased on CXR films. The PVMs are either decreased (asplenia) or increased (polysplenia). The heart is in the right or left chest or in the midline (mesocardia). A symmetric liver (midline liver) is a striking feature of both syndromes.

4. When the systematic approach is used, 2D echo and color flow Doppler studies can detect all or most of the anomalies described under pathology.

5. Laboratory findings
   a. Howell-Jolly and Heinz bodies seen on the peripheral smear suggest asplenia syndrome, although some normal newborns and septic infants may show these bodies.
   b. A splenic scan may be useful in differentiating the two conditions in older infants but is of limited value in acutely ill neonates.

6. Without palliative surgical procedures, more than 95% of patients with asplenia syndrome die in the first year of life. Fulminating sepsis is one of the causes of death. Excessive nodal bradycardia with resulting CHF may develop in patients with polysplenia syndrome, requiring a pacemaker therapy.

Management

Medical

a. PGE_1 infusion is indicated for severely cyanotic newborns with asplenia syndrome to reopen the ductus in preparation for an S-P shunt.

b. Patients with polysplenia syndrome may need treatment of CHF with anticongestive agents. Occasionally a PA banding is necessary if an intractable CHF develops with a large PBF.

c. For prevention of fulminating infections, continuous antibiotic therapy with amoxicillin (20 to 25 mg/kg/day in two divided doses) up to 2 years of age and immunization with polyvalent pneumococcal vaccine and quadrivalent meningococcal vaccine (at 2 years of age) and hemophilus B conjugate vaccine (in infancy, as for healthy children) are recommended for children with asplenia syndrome. Revaccination after 3 to 5 years should be considered for asplenia syndrome.

Surgical

a. An S-P shunt is usually necessary for newborns and infants with asplenia syndrome. Mortality is high, probably because of regurgitation of the common AV valve and undiagnosed obstructive TAPVR. In infants with infracardiac TAPVR, a successful connection can be made between the pulmonary venous confluence and the RA with the use of a partial exclusion clamp and without cardiopulmonary bypass.

b. Occasional patients with polysplenia syndrome require a PA banding for an intractable CHF.

c. For asplenia syndrome a Fontan-type operation can be performed (after the patient is age 3) but surgical mortality is as high as 65% (because of the AV valve regurgitation).

d. In some children with polysplenia syndrome, total correction of the defect is possible. If not, a Fontan operation can be performed, (with mortality of about 25%).

e. Occasionally pacemaker therapy is required for excessive junctional bradycardia and CHF in children with polysplenia syndrome.

IV. MISCELLANEOUS CONGENITAL ANOMALIES

A. Anomalous Origin of the Left Coronary Artery (Bland-White-Garland Syndrome, ALCAPA Syndrome)

The left coronary artery arises abnormally from the PA. The newborn patient is usually asymptomatic until the PA pressure falls to a critical level. Symptoms appear at 2 to 3 months of age and consist of recurring episodes of distress (anginal pain), marked cardiomegaly, and CHF. Heart murmur usually is absent. The ECG shows an anterolateral myocardial infarction pattern consisting of abnormally deep and wide Q waves, inverted T waves, and ST segment shift in leads I, aVL, and most precordial leads.

All such patients need surgery. The optimal operation in infancy remains controversial.

1. Palliative surgery: In critically ill infants, although less desirable than primary repair, simple ligation of the anomalous left coronary artery close to its origin from the PA may be carried out to prevent steal into the PA. This should be followed by an elective bypass procedure later.

2. Definitive surgery

   a. Intrapulmonary tunnel operation (Takeuchi repair) is most popular among two-coronary repair surgeries. A tunnel is created along the posterior wall of the PA using the flap of the anterior wall of the PA, which connects the opening of a surgically created aortopulmonary window and the orifice of the anomalous left coronary artery. Mortality ranges from none to as high as 40%. This procedure has the inherent disadvantage of late obstruction of the tunnel or obstruction to the MPA.

b. Left coronary artery implantation. Direct transfer of the anomalous left coronary artery into the aortic root appears to be the most desirable procedure but is not always possible.

c. Subclavian–left coronary artery anastomosis. The end of the left subclavian artery is turned down and anastomosed end to end to the anomalous left coronary artery.

d. In Tashiro procedure (1993), which was described in adults, a narrow cuff of the MPA, including the orifice of the left artery, is transected. The upper and lower edges of the cuff are closed to form a new left main coronary artery, which is anastomosed to the aorta. The divided MPA is anastomosed end to end.

B. Arteriovenous Fistula, Coronary

These fistulae occur in one of two patterns: They may represent a branching tributary from a coronary artery coursing along a normal anatomic distribution ("true coronary arteriovenous fistula), occuring in only 7% of patients. In most patients the fistula is the result of an abnormal coronary artery system with aberrant termination (coronary artery fistula). In most cases the fistula terminates in the right side of the heart (40% in the RV, 25% in the RA, and 20% in the PA).

The patient is usually asymptomatic. A continuous murmur similar to the murmur of PDA is audible over the precordium rather than in the left infraclavicular area. The ECG is usually normal, but it may show T wave inversion, RVH, or LVH if the fistula is large. CXR films usually show normal heart size. Bacterial endocarditis, fistula rupture, and myocardial infarction are significant risks.

In surgery the fistulous point is closed nearest to the entry into the cardiac chamber without compromising the coronary circulation (surgical mortality 0% to 5%). Recently, successful use of Gianturco coils or a double umbrella device has seen reported in selected patients.

C. Arteriovenous Fistula, Pulmonary

There is direct communication between the PAs and PVs, bypassing the pulmonary capillary circulation. They may take the form of either multiple tiny angiomas (telangiectasis) or a large PA-to-PV communication. About 60% of patients with pulmonary AV fistulas have Rendu-Osler-Weber syndrome. Rarely, chronic liver disease or a previous Fontan operation may cause the fistula.

Cyanosis and clubbing are present, with a varying degree of arterial saturation ranging from 50% to 85%. A faint systolic or continuous murmur may be audible over the affected area. The peripheral pulses are not bounding. Polycythemia is usually present, and arterial saturation runs between 50% and 85%. CXR films show normal heart size. One or more rounded opacities of variable size may be present in the lung fields. The ECG is usually normal. Stroke, brain abscess, rupture of the fistula with hemoptysis or hemothorax, and infective endocarditis are possible complications. The definitive diagnosis of the condition requires pulmonary angiography.

Surgical resection of the lesions, with preservation of as much healthy lung tissue as possible, may be attempted in symptomatic children, but the progressive nature of the disorder calls for a conservative approach. Recently, selective embolotherapy has been proposed as an alternative to surgical resection.

D. Arteriovenous Fistula, Systemic

There is a direct communication (either a vascular channel or angiomas) between the artery and vein without the interposition of the capillary bed. The two most common sites of systemic AV fistulae are the brain and liver. Because of decreased peripheral vascular resistance, an increase in stroke volume (with a wide pulse pressure), cardiomegaly, tachycardia, and even CHF result.

A systolic or continuous murmur is audible over the affected organ. A systolic ejection murmur may be audible as a result of increased blood flow through the semilunar valves. The peripheral pulses may be bounding during the high-output stage but weak if CHF develops. A gallop rhythm may be present with CHF. CXR films show cardiomegaly and increased PVMs. The ECG may show hypertrophy of either or both ventricles.

Most patients with large cerebral AV fistulae and CHF die as newborns, and surgical ligation of the affected artery to the brain is rarely possible without infarcting the brain. Surgical treatment of hepatic fistulae is often impossible because they are spread throughout the liver. Corticosteroids or radiotherapy may prove to be effective.

E. Cor Triatriatum

In this rare cardiac anomaly the LA is divided into two compartments by a fibromuscular septum with a small opening, producing obstruction of pulmonary venous return. Hemodynamic abnormalities of this condition are similar to those of MS in that both conditions produce pulmonary venous and arterial hypertension.

Important physical findings include dyspnea, basal pulmonary rales, a loud P2, and a nonspecific systolic murmur. The ECG shows RAD, severe RVH, and occasional RAH. CXR films show evidence of pulmonary venous congestion or pulmonary edema, prominent MPA segment, and right-sided heart enlargement. Echo demonstrates a linear structure within the LA cavity. Surgical correction is always indicated. Pulmonary hypertension regresses rapidly in survivors if the correction is made early.

F. Dextrocardia and Mesocardia

The terms *dextrocardia* (heart in the right side of the chest) and *mesocardia* (heart in midline of the thorax) express the position of the heart as a whole but do not specify the segmental relationship of the heart. A normally formed heart can be in the right chest because of extracardiac abnormalities. On the other hand, a heart in the right chest may be a sign of a serious cyanotic heart defect. The segmental approach is used to examine the significance of abnormal position of the heart.

The Segmental Approach

The heart and the great arteries can be viewed as three separate segments, the atria, the ventricles, and the great arteries. These three segments can vary from their normal positions either independently or together, resulting in many possible sets of abnormalities. Accurate mapping can be accomplished by echo and angiocardiography, but CXR and ECG are helpful also.

Localization of the Atria: Chest x-rays, the ECG, and the echo can be used to localize the atria.

1. CXR film
   a. Right-sided liver shadow and left-sided stomach bubble indicate situs solitus of the atria. Left-sided liver shadow and right-sided stomach bubble indicate situs inversus of the atria.
   b. A midline (symmetric) liver shadow on CXR film suggests splenic syndromes in which either two right atria or two left atria are present with associated complex cardiac anomalies (see Splenic Syndromes).
2. ECG: The SA node is always located in the RA. Therefore, the P axis of the ECG can be used to locate the atria. When the P axis is in the left lower quadrant (0 to +90 degrees), situs solitus of the atria is present. When the P axis is in the right lower quadrant (+90 to +180 degrees), situs inversus of the atria is present. With splenic syndromes, the P axis may be superiorly directed (polysplenia syndrome) or may change between the left lower quadrant and the right lower quadrant from time to time (asplenia syndrome).
3. 2D echo: The 2D echo identifies the IVC and/or pulmonary veins. The RA is connected to the IVC, and the LA receives the pulmonary veins.

Localization of the Ventricles: Ventricular localization can be accomplished noninvasively by the ECG and 2D echo.

1. ECG: The depolarization of the ventricular septum takes place from the embryonic LV to the RV, producing Q waves in the precordial leads that lie over

the anatomic LV. If Q waves are present in V5 and V6 as well as lead I but not in V1, D-loop of the ventricle as in normal persons is likely. If Q waves are present in V4R, V1, and V2 but not in V5 and V6, L-loop of the ventricles is likely (ventricular inversion, as seen in L-TGA).

2. 2D echo: The tricuspid valve leaflet usually inserts on the interventricular septum in a more apical position than does the mitral septal leaflet. The RV is attached to the tricuspid valve. The LV has two papillary muscles.

Localization of the Great Arteries: The ECG is not helpful in finding the great arteries; 2D echo studies can locate them accurately.

Types of Displacement: The four most common types of dextrocardia are classic mirror-image dextrocardia, normal heart displaced to the right side of the chest, congenitally corrected TGA, and single ventricle (Fig 3-18). Less commonly, asplenia and polysplenia syndromes with situs ambiguus and complicated cardiac defects cause dextrocardia. All of these abnormalities may result in mesocardia. With CXR films and ECGs the segmental approach discussed earlier can be used to deduce the nature of segmental relationship in dextrocardia, as well as in mesocardia.

1. Classic mirror-image dextrocardia (Fig 3-18, A) shows the liver shadow on the left on CXR films. The ECG shows the P axis between +90 and +180 degrees and Q waves in V5R and V6R.

2. Normally formed heart shifted toward the right side of the chest (dextroversion) (Fig 3-18, B) shows the liver shadow on the right on CXR films, the P axis between 0 and +90 degrees, and Q waves in V5 and V6 on the ECG.

3. Congenitally corrected L-TGA with situs solitus (Fig 3-18, C) shows situs solitus of abdominal viscera on CXR films. The ECG shows the P axis in the normal quadrant (0 to +90 degrees) and Q waves in V5R and V6R.

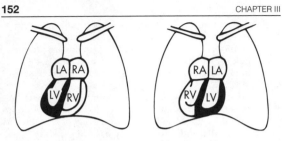

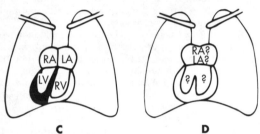

FIG. 3-18.
Examples of common conditions when the apex of the heart is in the right side of the chest. (From Park MK, Guntheroth WG: *How to Read Pediatric ECGs,* ed 3, St. Louis, Mosby, 1992.)

4. Undifferentiated cardiac chambers (Fig 3-18, *D*) are often associated with complicated cardiac defects and may show midline liver on CXR films. The ECG may show shifting or superiorly oriented P axis and abnormal Q waves in the precordial leads.

G. Systemic Venous Anomalies

There are wide ranges of abnormalities of the systemic venous system, some of which have little physiological importance. Others have surgical significance or produce cyanosis. Two well-known anomalies of systemic veins are persistent left SVC and infrahepatic interruption of the IVC with azygos continuation. Rarely either persistent left SVC or interrupted IVC can drain into the LA, producing cyanosis.

Anomalies of Superior Vena Cava

1. Persistent left SVC draining into the RA. In the most commonly encountered type, the left SVC is connected to the coronary sinus (Fig 3-19, *A*). As a rule, persistent left SVC is part of a bilateral SVC, but rarely the right SVC is absent (Fig 3-19, *B*). A bridging innominate vein is present in 60% of cases.

   Isolated persistent left SVC does not produce symptoms or signs. Cardiac examination is entirely normal. CXR films may show the shadow of the left SVC along the left upper border of the mediastinum. There is a high prevalence of leftward P axis (+15 degrees or less) on the ECG. The enlarged coronary sinus may be imaged by an echo study. Treatment for isolated persistent left SVC is not necessary.

2. Persistent left SVC draining into the LA (Fig 3-19, *C*, *D*). Rarely, because of the absence of the coronary sinus, persistent left SVC drains into the LA (8% of cases) resulting in systemic arterial desaturation. Associated cardiac anomalies, usually of complex cyanotic type, are almost invariably present. Defects of the atrial septum (single atrium, secundum ASD, primum ASD) are also frequently found. Clinical manifestations are dominated by the associated complex cardiac defects. Surgical correction is necessary.

Anomalies of the Inferior Vena Cava

1. Interrupted IVC with azygos continuation (Fig 3-20, *A*) has been reported in about 3% of children with CHDs. Instead of receiving the hepatic veins and entering the RA, the IVC drains via an enlarged azygos system into the right SVC and eventually to the RA. The hepatic veins connect directly to the RA. Bilateral SVC is also common. Azygos continuation of the IVC is often associated with various types of complex cyanotic heart defects. No case has been re-

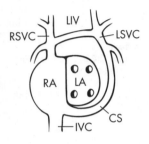
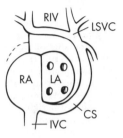

A   **B**

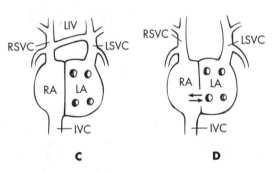

C   **D**

FIG. 3-19.
Schematic diagram of Persistent LSVC. **A,** LSVC drains via CS into
the RA. The LIV and the RSVC are adequate. **B,** Uncommonly, the
RSVC may be atretic. The CS is large because it receives blood from
both the right and left upper parts of the body. **C,** The coronary sinus
is absent and LSVC drains directly into the LA. The atrial septum is
intact. **D,** The LSVC connects to the LA, and a posterior ASD allows
a predominant left-to-right atrial shunt. *LSVC,* left superior vena
cava; *CS,* coronary sinus; *LIV,* left innominate vein.

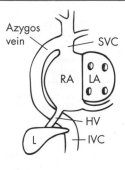

A

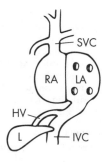

B

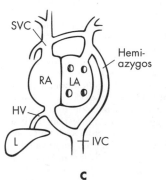

C

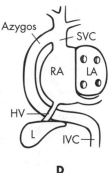

D

FIG. 3-20.

Schematic diagram of selected abnormalities of the IVC. **A,** Interrupted IVC with azygos continuation, the most common abnormality of the IVC. The HV connect directly to the RA. **B,** Right IVC draining into the LA. **C,** Absence of the lower right IVC. The IVC drains into LSVC and LA and to the RA through the hepatic portion of the IVC. **D,** Complete absence of the right IVC with communicating vein draining to the azygos vein. *HV,* hepatic veins.

ported in association with asplenia syndrome. This defect creates difficulties during cardiac catheterization and can render surgical correction of an underlying cardiac defect more difficult. There is no need for surgical correction of this venous anomaly per se.

2. IVC connecting to the LA is an extremely rare condition in which the IVC receives the hepatic veins, curves toward the LA, and makes a direct connection with the chamber (Fig 3-20, *B*), producing cyanosis. Surgical correction is indicated.

H. Vascular Ring

Prevalence: Vascular ring reportedly constitutes fewer than 1% of all congenital cardiovascular anomalies, but this is probably an underestimation.

Pathology: Vascular ring is a group of anomalies of the aortic arch that cause respiratory symptoms or feeding problems. The vascular ring may be complete (true) or incomplete.

1. In complete vascular ring the abnormal vascular structures form a complete circle around the trachea and esophagus. These include double aortic arch and right aortic arch with left ligamentum arteriosum.

2. Incomplete vascular ring comprises vascular anomalies that do not form a complete circle around the trachea and esophagus but do compress the trachea or esophagus. These include anomalous innominate artery, aberrant right subclavian artery, and anomalous left pulmonary artery (vascular sling).

Clinical Manifestations: Respiratory distress and feeding problems of varying severity appear at varying ages. History of pneumonia is frequently elicited. Physical examination is not revealing except for varying degrees of rhonchi. Cardiac examination and the ECG are normal. CXR films may reveal compression of the air-filled trachea. Aspiration pneumonia or atelectasis may be present. Barium esophagogram is usually diagnostic except in anomalous innominate artery (Fig 3-21). Angiography is usually indicated to confirm the diagnosis and to prepare for surgery.

	Anatomy	Ba-Esophagogram	Other X-ray findings	Symptoms	Treatment
Double aortic arch	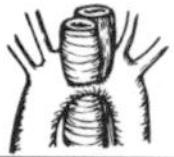	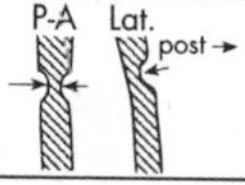	Anterior compression of trachea	Respiratory difficulty (onset < 3 mo) Swallowing dysfunction	Surgical division of a smaller arch
Right aortic arch with left ligamentum arteriosum	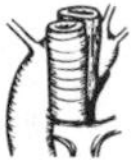	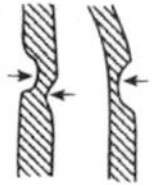		Mild respiratory difficulty (onset > 1 year) Swallowing dysfunction	Surgical division of the ligamentum arteriosum
Anomalous innominate artery	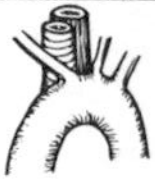	Normal	Anterior compression of trachea	Stridor and/or cough in infancy	Conservative management or surgical suturing of the artery to the sternum
Aberrant right subclavian artery	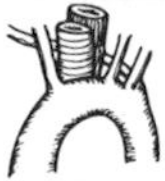	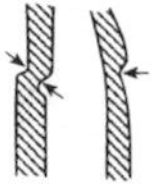		Occasional swallowing dysfunction	Usually no treatment
Vascular sling	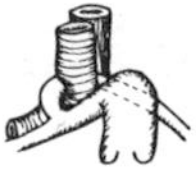	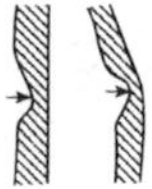	Right-sided emphysema or atelectasis; posterior compression of trachea or right main stem bronchus	Wheezing and cyanotic episodes since birth	Surgical division of the anomalous LPA (from the RPA) and anastomosis to the MPA

FIG. 3-21.
Summary and clinical features of vascular ring. *P-A*, posteroanterior view; *Lat*, lateral view.

Management: Medical management is indicated for infants with mild symptoms. A surgical approach is indicated for infants with more severe symptoms or complications such as aspiration pneumonia (Fig 3-21).

ACQUIRED HEART DISEASE

IV

I. PRIMARY MYOCARDIAL DISEASE (CARDIOMYOPATHY)

Primary myocardial disease affects the heart muscle itself and is not associated with congenital, valvular, or coronary heart disease or systemic disorders. Cardiomyopathy has been classified into three types based on anatomic and functional features: (1) hypertrophic, (2) dilated (or congestive), and (3) restrictive (Fig 4-1). The three types of cardiomyopathies are functionally different from one another, and the demands of therapy are also different.

In *hypertrophic* cardiomyopathy there is a massive ventricular hypertrophy with an enhanced ventricular contractility, but ventricular filling is impaired due to relaxation abnormalities.

Dilated cardiomyopathy is characterized by a ventricular dilatation with a decreased contractile function. Endocardial fibroelastosis and doxorubicin cardiomyopathy have clinical features similar to those of dilated cardiomyopathy.

Restrictive cardiomyopathy denotes a restriction to diastolic ventricular filling caused by endocardial or myocardial disease (usually because of infiltrative disease), and contractile function of the ventricle may be normal.

A. Hypertrophic Cardiomyopathy

Pathology and Pathophysiology

1. A massive ventricular hypertrophy is present.
   Although asymmetric septal hypertrophy (ASH), formerly known as idiopathic hypertrophic subaortic ste-

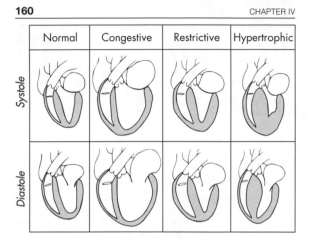

FIG. 4-1.
Diagram of 50-degree left anterior oblique view of heart in different
types of cardiomyopathy at end systole and end diastole. *Congestive* corresponds to *dilated* cardiomyopathy as used in the text.
(From Goldman MR, Boucher CA: Values of radionuclide imaging
techniques in assessing cardiomyopathy. Am J Cardiol 46:1232-1236, 1980.)

  nosis (IHSS), is the most common type, a concentric
hypertrophy with symmetric thickening of the LV
sometimes occurs. Occasionally an intracavitary obstruction may develop during systole, partly because
of systolic anterior motion (SAM) of the mitral valve
against the hypertrophied septum, called hypertrophic obstructive cardiomyopathy (HOCM).
2. The myocardium itself has an enhanced contractile
state, but diastolic ventricular filling is impaired because of abnormal stiffness of the LV. This may lead
to LA enlargement and pulmonary venous congestion, producing congestive symptoms (exertional dyspnea, orthopnea, paroxysmal nocturnal dyspnea).

Clinical Manifestations

1. Some 30% to 60% of cases are seen in adolescents and young adults with positive family history. Easy fatigability, dyspnea, palpitation, or anginal pain may be the presenting complaint.

2. A sharp upstroke of the arterial pulse is characteristic. A late systolic ejection murmur of medium pitch, best audible at the middle and lower LSB or at the apex, is usually heard. A holosystolic murmur of MR is occasionally present. The intensity and even the presence of the heart murmur vary from examination to examination.

3. The ECG may show LVH, ST-T changes, abnormally deep Q waves with diminished or absent R waves in the LPLs, and arrhythmias.

4. CXR films may show mild LV enlargement with globular heart.

5. Echo demonstrates hypertrophy of the septum (ASH) and/or the LV free wall. In obstructive type, SAM of the mitral valve may be demonstrated. The Doppler examination of the mitral inflow demonstrates a decreased E velocity, an increased A velocity, and a decreased E/A ratio.

6. The obstruction may be absent, stable, or slowly progressive. Sudden death may occur, particularly during exercise.

Management

1. Moderate restriction of physical activity is recommended.

2. A β-adrenergic blocker (such as propranolol, atenolol, or metoprolol) is the drug of choice in the obstructive subgroup. These drugs reduce the degree of obstruction, decrease the incidence of anginal pain, and have antiarrhythmic actions. Calcium channel blockers, principally verapamil, may be equally effective. Prophylactic therapy with either β-adrenergic blockers or verapamil is controversial.

3. Digitalis, other cardiotonic drugs, and vasodilators are contraindicated, as they increase the degree of obstruction.

4. SBE prophylaxis should be observed if indicated.
5. Transaortic left ventricular septal myotomy and myectomy (Morrow myectomy) may be indicated in selected symptomatic patients who are not responding to medical management. Rarely, mitral valve replacement may be indicated.

B. Dilated (Congestive) Cardiomyopathy

Pathology and Pathophysiology: In dilated cardiomyopathy a weakening of systolic contraction is associated with dilatation of all four cardiac chambers. Intracavitary thrombus formation is common in the apical portion of the ventricular cavities and in atrial appendages, and it may give rise to pulmonary and systemic embolization. Dilated cardiomyopathy may be the end result of myocardial damage produced by a variety of infectious, toxic, or metabolic agents or immunologic defects.

Clinical Manifestations

1. Fatigue, weakness, and symptoms of left heart failure (e.g., dyspnea on exertion, orthopnea) may be present.
2. Signs of CHF (e.g., tachycardia, pulmonary rales, weak pulses, distended neck veins, hepatomegaly) may be present. A prominent S3 with or without gallop rhythm is present. A soft systolic murmur of MR or TR may be present.
3. Sinus tachycardia, LVH, and ST-T changes are common ECG findings.
4. CXR films show generalized cardiomegaly, often with signs of pulmonary venous congestion.
5. Echo is diagnostic. The LV and RV are dilated with a reduced fractional shortening (FS) and ejection fraction (EF). Intracavitary thrombus and pericardial effusion may be present. The mitral inflow Doppler tracing demonstrates a reduced E velocity and a decreased E/A ratio.
6. Progressive deterioration is the rule rather than the exception. About two thirds of these patients die within 4 years of the onset of symptoms, of

arrhythmias, systemic or pulmonary embolization, or CHF.

Management

1. CHF is treated with digoxin, diuretics, vasodilators (captopril, enalapril, hydralazine), bed rest, and restriction of activity.
2. Anticoagulation (coumadin or heparin) is recommended because of the frequency of embolization.
3. Arrhythmias may be treated with amiodarone, other antiarrhythmic agents, or a pacemaker.
4. Beneficial effects of β-adrenergic blockers (somewhat heretical given poor LV contractility) is under investigation.
5. Cardiac transplantation may be indicated.

C. Endocardial Fibroelastosis

Pathology: Endocardial fibroelastosis (EFE) is a form of dilated cardiomyopathy of unknown origin seen in infants and children. The condition is characterized by diffuse changes in the endocardium with a white, opaque, glistening appearance. The left side of the heart is dilated and hypertrophied with poor contractility. For unknown reasons the incidence of EFE has declined in the past 2 decades.

Clinical Manifestations

1. Symptoms and signs of CHF develop in the first 10 months of life.
2. No heart murmur is audible in most patients, although gallop rhythm is usually present. Occasionally a heart murmur of MR is audible. Hepatomegaly is usually present.
3. The ECG shows LVH with strain. Occasionally myocardial infarction patterns and arrhythmias are seen.
4. CXR films show marked cardiomegaly with normal PVMs or pulmonary venous congestion patterns.

Treatment: Early and long-term (years) treatment with digoxin, diuretics, and afterload-reducing agents is recommended. With proper treatment about a third of the patients recover completely. Another third do not improve, and the remaining third gradually deteriorate and die.

D. Doxorubicin Cardiomyopathy

Etiology and Pathology: Doxorubicin cardiomyopathy is becoming the most common cause of chronic CHF in children. Risk factors include (1) age younger than 4 years, (2) the cumulative dose exceeding 400 to 600 mg/m^2, and (3) a regimen of larger, infrequent doses. It occurrs in up to 50% of patients who have received more than $1\ g/m^2$ of doxorubicin. A dilated LV with decreased contractility and elevated filling pressures and reduced cardiac output characterize pathophysiologic features.

Clinical Manifestations

1. Patients are usually asymptomatic until signs of CHF develop. Symptoms may develop 2 to 4 months, and rarely, years, after completion of doxorubicin therapy. History of exertional dyspnea, palpitation, cough, or substernal discomfort may be present.
2. Signs of CHF develop with hepatomegaly and distended neck veins. Gallop rhythm may be audible with occasional soft systolic murmur of MR or TR.
3. CXR films show cardiomegaly with or without pulmonary congestion or pleural effusion.
4. The ECG shows sinus tachycardia with rare ST-T changes.
5. Echo studies reveal a dilated LV with decreased contractility.
6. Symptomatic cardiomyopathy carries a high mortality rate. The 2-year survival rate is about 20%, and almost all patients die by 9 years after onset of the illness.

Management

1. Anticongestive measures with inotropic agents (digoxin), diuretics, and after-load-reducing agents (captopril) are useful.
2. Doxorubicin administered as a continuous infusion can reduce cardiac injury.

3. The advisability of the modification of anthracycline therapy is controversial. The Cardiology Committee of Children's Cancer Study Group (Pediatrics 89:942-949, 1992) has recommended close monitoring for cardiac toxicity by echo, radionuclide angiography, and endomyocardial biopsy, and if these tests show abnormalities of LV systolic function, either withholding anthracycline therapy (limiting the total cumulative dose to 400 to 500 mg/m^2) or reducing the subsequent dose. Others recommend dose modification only when clinical evidence of cardiotoxicity is present.

4. Cardiac transplantation may be an option for selected patients.

E. Restrictive Cardiomyopathy

1. The least common of the three types of cardiomyopathy is characterized by an abnormal diastolic ventricular filling owing to excessively stiff ventricular walls, often caused by infiltrative disease processes (e.g., sarcoidosis, amyloidosis). The ventricles remain normal in size and maintain normal contractility, but the atria are enlarged out of proportion to the ventricles. Endomyocardial biopsy may be useful in identifying causes of restrictive cardiomyopathies (e.g., amyloidosis, hemochromatosis, glycogen deposit).

2. History of exercise intolerance, weakness and dyspnea, or chest pain may be present. Jugular venous distention, gallop rhythm, and a systolic murmur of MR or TR may be present. CXR films show cardiomegaly, pulmonary congestion, and pleural effusion. The ECG may show atrial fibrillation and paroxysms of SVT. Echo studies reveal characteristic biatrial enlargement, with normal cavity size of the LV and RV. LV systolic function (ejection fraction) is normal until the late stages of the disease. Atrial thrombus may be present. The mitral inflow Doppler tracing shows an increased E velocity and increased E/A ratio.

3. Diuretics are beneficial (but digoxin is not indicated, since systolic function is unimpaired). Anticoagulants (warfarin) and antiplatelet drugs (aspirin and di-

pyridamole) may help prevent thrombosis. Corticosteroids and immunosuppressive agents have been
suggested. Permanent pacemaker is indicated for
complete heart block, and cardiac transplantation
may be an option.

F. Right Ventricular Dysplasia

1. RV dysplasia, or RV cardiomyopathy, is a rare abnormality of unknown etiology in which the myocardium
   of the RV is partially or totally replaced by fibrous or
   adipose tissue. The LV is usually spared. Most cases
   appear to be sporadic. It is prevalent in northern
   Italy.
2. The onset is in infancy, childhood, or adulthood
   (but usually before age 20), with history of palpitation, syncopal episodes, or both. Sudden death
   may be the first sign of the disease. Presenting
   manifestations may be arrhythmias (ventricular
   tachycardia, supraventricular arrhythmias), or signs
   of CHF. CXR films usually show cardiomegaly, and
   the ECG most often shows tall P waves in lead II
   (RAH) and decreased RV potentials. Echo shows
   selective RV enlargement and often areas of akine-
   sia or dyskinesia.
3. A substantial portion of patients die before age 5 of
   CHF and intractable ventricular tachycardia. Various
   antiarrhythmic agents may be tried, but they are often
   unsuccessful in abolishing ventricular tachycardia.
   Surgical intervention (ventricular incision or discon-
   nection of the RV free wall) may be tried if antiarrhythmic therapy is unsuccessful.

II. CARDIOVASCULAR INFECTIONS

A. Infective Endocarditis (Subacute Bacterial Endocarditis)

Prevalence: Subacute bacterial endocarditis (SBE) affects 0.5:1000 to 1:1000 hospital patients, excluding
those with postoperative endocarditis.

Pathogenesis and Pathology

1. Two factors are important in the pathogenesis of infective endocarditis: (1) structural abnormalities of the heart or great arteries with a significant pressure gradient or turbulence with resulting endothelial damage and platelet-fibrin thrombus formation, and (2) bacteremia, even if transient. Bacteremia frequently results from dental procedures and chewing with diseased teeth.

2. All CHDs (except secundum ASD) and valvular heart diseases predispose to endocarditis. Those with a prosthetic heart valve or prosthetic material in the heart are at particularly high risk for infective endocarditis. Drug addicts may develop endocarditis in the absence of known cardiac anomalies.

3. *Streptococcus viridans, Streptococcus faecalis* (enterococcus), and *Staphylococcus aureus* are responsible for more than 90% of cases.

Clinical Manifestations

1. Underlying heart defect is present in almost all patients. History of recent dental procedures, tonsillectomy, or toothache is common. The onset of the illness is insidious, with fever, fatigue, loss of appetite, and pallor.

2. Heart murmur and fever are almost always present. Splenomegaly is common (70% of patients).

3. Skin manifestations (seen in 50% of patients), probably secondary to microemboli, may include petechiae, Osler nodes (tender red nodes at the ends of the fingers), Janeway lesions (small, painless hemorrhagic areas on the palms or soles), and splinter hemorrhage (linear hemorrhagic streaks beneath the nails).

4. Embolic phenomena to other organs (e.g. pulmonary emboli, seizures and hemiparesis, hematuria) affect 50% of patients.

5. Carious teeth or periodontal or gingival disease is frequently present.

6. Positive blood cultures, anemia, leukocytosis, and increased erythrocyte sedimentation rate (ESR) are the key laboratory findings.

7. 2D echo may actually demonstrate the vegetation. It is unlikely that vegetations less than 2 mm in maximum dimension will be imaged by 2D echo.

Diagnosis: A presumptive diagnosis of infective endocarditis is made when a patient with an underlying heart lesion has a fever of unknown origin of several days' duration and any of the typical physical findings or laboratory changes is present. A definitive diagnosis is made by positive blood culture. Demonstration of the vegetation by 2D echo is a conclusive anatomic diagnosis.

Management

1. Four to six blood cultures are obtained in succession over 24 to 48 hours.

2. IV penicillin or oxacillin plus IV gentamicin or IM streptomycin are started pending the results of blood cultures.
   a. Penicillin G 200,000 U/kg/day (maximum 20 million U/day) IV bolus in six divided doses.
   b. Oxacillin 150 to 200 mg/kg/day (maximum 12 g/day) IV bolus in six divided doses.
   c. Gentamicin 7 mg/kg/day (maximum 240 mg/day) IV in three divided doses.
   d. Streptomycin 30 mg/kg/day (maximum 1 g/day) IM in one or two divided doses.

3. Final selection of antibiotics depends on the organism isolated and the result of antibiotic sensitivity test. Penicillin-allergic individuals may be treated with IV vancomycin 40 mg/kg/day (maximum of 2 g/day) in four divided doses. The duration of treatment is 4 to 6 weeks.

4. Operative intervention may be necessary before the antibiotic therapy is complete if the clinical situation warrants (e.g., progressive CHF, significant malfunction of prosthetic valves, persistently positive blood cultures after 2 weeks' therapy). Bacteriologic relapse after an appropriate course of therapy also calls for operative intervention.

Prognosis: The overall recovery rate is 80% to 85%. The recovery rate for streptococcal and enterococcal endocarditis is better than 90%.

Prevention: Good dental hygiene is more important than antibiotic prophylaxis. Antibiotic prophylaxis for endocarditis is recommended only for patients having certain cardiac conditions and procedures (Table 4-1). The "Prevention of Bacterial Endocarditis" wallet card (based on recommendations of the American Heart Association, December 1990) is reproduced in the Appendix, Figure A-1.

B. Myocarditis

Etiology: Myocarditis may be caused by an infectious agent, immune mediated process, collagen disease or toxic agent. A cell-mediated immunologic reaction, not merely myocardial damage from viral replication, appears important in viral myocarditis.

1. Infections: Viruses are probably the most common cause of myocarditis in North America; coxsackieviruses and echoviruses are the most common agents. Many other viruses (such as poliomyelitis, mumps, measles, rubella, cytomegalovirus, HIV, arboviruses, adenovirus, and influenza) can cause myocarditis. In South America Chaga disease (caused by *Trypanosoma cruzi*, a protozoon) is far more common. Rarely, bacteria, rickettsia, fungi, protozoa, and parasites are the causative agents.
2. Immune mediated diseases: acute rheumatic fever, Kawasaki disease.
3. Collagen vascular diseases.
4. Toxic myocarditis (drug ingestion, diphtheria exotoxin, and anoxic agents).

Clinical Manifestations

1. History of an upper respiratory infection may be present in older children. The onset of illness may be sudden in newborns and small infants, causing anorexia, vomiting, lethargy, and occasionally circulatory shock.
2. Signs of CHF (e.g., poor heart tone, tachycardia, gallop rhythm, tachypnea, hepatomegaly, and rarely, cyanosis) may be present. A soft systolic heart murmur may be audible. An irregular rhythm caused by supraventricular or ventricular ectopic beats may be present.

TABLE 4-1.

Indications and Nonindications for Infective Endocarditis Prophylaxis

---

Indications for Prophylaxis

Conditions

Most congenital heart defects

Rheumatic and other valvular diseases

Hypertrophic cardiomyopathy

MVP with MR

Prosthetic cardiac valves, including bioprosthetic and homograft valves

Systemic-pulmonary artery shunts

History of infective endocarditis, even in the absence of heart disease

Procedures

Dental procedures known to induce gingival or mucosal bleeding, including routine professional dental cleaning

Tonsillectomy and adenoidectomy, surgical procedures of respiratory tract, bronchoscopy with a rigid bronchoscope

Esophageal dilation

Gallbladder or gastrointestinal surgery

Urethral dilation, cystoscopy, urethral catheterization or urinary tract surgery associated with urinary tract infection, prostatic surgery

Incision and drainage of infected tissue

Vaginal hysterectomy and vaginal delivery in the presence of infection

---

Not Indications for Prophylaxis

Conditions

Isolated secundum ASD

Surgical repair without residua beyond 6 months of secundum ASD, VSD or PDA

Previous coronary artery bypass surgery

MVP without MR

Innocent heart murmurs

Previous Kawasaki disease without valvular dysfunction

Previous rheumatic fever without valvular disease

Cardiac pacemakers and implanted defibrillators

TABLE 4-1.

Indications and Nonindications for Infective Endocarditis
Prophylaxis—cont'd

Procedures

Shedding of primary teeth, simple adjustment of orthodontic
   appliances, filling above the gum line, injection of intraoral
   anesthetic
Tympanostomy tube insertion
Endotracheal intubation, bronchoscopy with a flexible bronchoscope with or without biopsy
Cardiac catheterization
Endoscopy with or without gastrointestinal biopsy
Cesarean section
(In the absence of infection), urethral catheterization, dilatation
   and curettage, uncomplicated vaginal delivery, therapeutic
   abortion, sterilization procedures, insertion or removal of
   intrauterine devices

---

3. The ECG may show any one or combination of the
   following: low QRS voltages, ST-T changes, prolongation of the QT interval, and arrhythmias, especially
   premature contractions.
4. Cardiomegaly on CXR films is the most important
   clinical sign of myocarditis.
5. Echo reveals cardiac chamber enlargement and
   impaired LV function, often regional. Occasionally, increased wall thickness and LV thrombi are
   found.
6. Radionuclide scanning (after the administration of
   gallium-67 or technetium-99m pyrophosphate) may
   identify inflammatory and necrotic changes characteristic of myocarditis.
7. The majority of patients, especially those with only
   mild inflammation, recover completely. Some patients
   develop subacute or chronic myocarditis with persistent cardiomegaly, with or without signs of CHF, and
   ECG evidence of LVH or CVH. Clinically, these patients are indistinguishable from those with dilated
   cardiomyopathy or endocardial fibroeleastosis.

Management

1. Virus identification by viral cultures from the blood, stool, or throat washing should be attempted, and comparison of acute and convalescent sera may be made for serologic titer rise.

2. Bed rest and limitation of activities are recommended during the acute phase (since exercise intensifies the damage from myocarditis in experimental animals).

3. Anticongestive measures include rapid-acting diuretics (e.g., furosemide or ethacrynic acid), rapid-acting inotropic agents (e.g., isoproterenol, dobutamine, or dopamine), administration of oxygen and bed rest. Cardiac chair or infant seat may be used for infants to relieve respiratory distress. Digoxin may be given cautiously, using half of the usual digitalizing dose, as some patients with myocarditis are exquisitely sensitive to it. An ACE inhibitor (e.g., captopril) may prove beneficial in the acute phase (as demonstrated in animal experiments).

4. Beneficial effects of high-dose γ-globulin (2 g/kg over 24 hours) have recently been reported (with better survival and better LV function by echo). A high dose of γ-globulin is an immunomodulatory agent, shown to be effective in myocarditis secondary to Kawasaki disease.

5. The role of corticosteroids is unclear except for the treatment of severe rheumatic carditis.

6. Specific therapies: Antitoxin in diphtheric myocarditis; γ-globulin and salicylates in Kawasaki myocarditis.

C. Pericarditis

Etiology

1. Viral infection is probably the most common cause, particularly in infancy.

2. Acute rheumatic fever is a common cause of pericarditis in certain parts of the world.

3. Bacterial infection (purulent pericarditis). Commonly encountered are *S. aureus, Streptococcus pneumoniae, Haemophilus influenzae, Neisseria meningitidis,* and streptococci.

4. Tuberculosis (an occasional cause of constrictive pericarditis with insidious onset).
5. Heart surgery (postpericardiotomy syndrome; see Chapter 8).
6. Collagen disease such as rheumatoid arthritis.
7. A complication of oncologic disease or its therapy, including radiation.
8. Uremia (uremic pericarditis).

Pathophysiology

1. Pathogenesis of symptoms and signs of pericardial effusion is determined by two factors: speed of fluid accumulation and competence of the myocardium. A rapid accumulation of a large amount of fluid or a slow accumulation of a small amount of fluid in the presence of myocarditis can produce circulatory embarrassment. Slow accumulation of a large amount of fluid may be well tolerated if the myocardium is intact.
2. With the development of pericardial tamponade, these compensatory mechanisms are called upon: systemic and pulmonary venous constriction (to improve diastolic filling), an increase in the SVR (to raise falling blood pressure), and tachycardia (to improve cardiac output).

Clinical Manifestations

1. The patient may have a history of upper respiratory tract infection. Precordial pain (dull, aching, or stabbing) with occasional radiation to the shoulder and neck may be a presenting complaint. The pain may be relieved by leaning forward and made worse by supine position or deep inspiration.
2. Pericardial friction rub is the cardinal physical sign. The heart is hypodynamic, and heart murmur is usually absent, although it may be present in acute rheumatic fever. In children with purulent pericarditis, septic fever (101° to 105°F, or 38° to 41°C), tachycardia, chest pain, and dyspnea are almost always present. Signs of cardiac tamponade may be present (distant heart sounds, tachycardia, pulsus paradoxus,

hepatomegaly, venous distention, and occasional hypotension with peripheral vasoconstriction).

3. The ECG may show a low-voltage QRS complex, ST segment shift, and T wave inversion.

4. CXR films may show a varying degree of cardiomegaly. Water bottle–shaped heart and increased pulmonary venous markings are seen with large effusion.

5. Echo is the most useful tool in establishing the diagnosis of pericardial effusion and in detecting cardiac tamponade (collapse of the RA or the RV free wall in diastole).

Management

1. Pericardiocentesis or surgical drainage to identify the cause of the pericarditis is mandatory, especially when purulent or tuberculous disease is suspected.

2. Salicylates may be administered for precordial pain in nonbacterial pericarditis and rheumatic fever. Corticosteroid therapy may be indicated for children with severe rheumatic carditis or postpericardiotomy syndrome.

3. For cardiac tamponade urgent decompression by surgical drainage or pericardiocentesis is indicated. While preparing for pericardial drainage, fluid push with plasmanate to increase central venous pressure is indicated to improve cardiac filling. Digitalis is contraindicated in cardiac tamponade (since it blocks tachycardia, the compensatory response to impaired venous return).

4. Urgent surgical drainage is indicated when purulent pericarditis is suspected. Purulent pericarditis is treated with an IV antibiotic therapy for 4 to 6 weeks.

D. Constrictive Pericarditis

1. A fibrotic, thickened, and adherent pericardium restricts diastolic filling of the heart. Although rare in children, it may be associated with earlier idiopathic or viral pericarditis, tuberculosis, incomplete drainage of purulent pericarditis, hemopericardium, mediastinal irradiation, neoplastic infiltration, or connective tissue disorders.

2. Diagnosis of constrictive pericarditis is suggested by the following clinical findings: signs of elevated jugular venous pressure; hepatomegaly with ascites and systemic edema; diastolic pericardial knock; calcification of the pericardium, enlargement of the SVC and the LA, and pleural effusion on CXR films; low QRS voltages, T wave inversion or flattening, LAH, and atrial fibrillation on the ECG.

3. An M-mode echo may reveal two parallel lines representing the thickened visceral and parietal pericardia or multiple dense echoes. Also, 2D echo shows an immobile and dense appearance of the pericardium, abrupt displacement of the interventricular septum during early diastolic filling (septal bounce), and dilatation of the hepatic veins and IVC. Cardiac catheterization may document constrictive physiology.

4. The treatment for constrictive pericarditis is complete resection of the pericardium; symptomatic improvement occurs in 75% of the patients.

III. KAWASAKI DISEASE (MUCOCUTANEOUS LYMPH NODE SYNDROME)

Etiology and Epidemiology

1. The cause of this disease is not known. It may be related to an infectious disease and abnormalities of the immune system initiated by the infectious insult. An environmental factor, such as toxin (rug or carpet cleaning), may also be important.

2. Children of all racial and ethnic groups are affected, although it is most common in Asians. It peaks in winter and spring. It occurs primarily in young children; 80% of the patients are younger than age 4, 50% are younger than age 2, and cases in children older than 8 years are rarely reported.

Pathology: This generalized febrile illness is accompanied by significant pathologies of the heart. There is vasculitis of the coronary artery with aneurysm formation that may lead to scar formation and calcification

TABLE 4-2.

Diagnostic Criteria for Kawasaki Disease

---

1. Fever, spiking up to 40° C (104° F), persisting for more than 5 days
2. Bilateral conjunctival injection without exudate
3. Changes in the mouth and lips: strawberry tongue, diffuse reddening of oral cavity, and erythema and cracking of the lips
4. Changes in the hands and feet: erythema and edema of the hands and feet
5. Polymorphous exanthem
6. Cervical lymphadenopathy greater than 1.5 cm in diameter, usually unilateral

---

When fever and four of the other five criteria are present, Kawasaki disease is probable. Coronary artery pathology may be diagnostic even when fewer than four criteria are present.

of the artery. Occasionally myocardial infarction leads to death. The elevated platelet count seen in this condition contributes to coronary thrombosis.

Clinical Manifestations

1. The clinical course of the disease may be divided into three phases; acute, subacute, and convalescent. Each phase of the disease is characterized by unique symptoms and signs.
   a. Acute phase (first 10 days)
      1) Six signs, the diagnostic criteria for Kawasaki disease, are present (Table 4-2).
      2) Other frequently associated findings include sterile pyuria (70%), arthritis (40%), gastrointestinal symptoms, hydrops of the gall bladder (25%), and aseptic meningitis (in almost all patients). Occasionally, a distinctive perineal rash develops 3 or 4 days from the onset of the illness; it desquamates in all instances by day 5 to 7.
      3) Cardiovascular abnormalities, which are most common during the subacute phase, may appear during the acute phase.

   b. Subacute phase (11 to 25 days after onset)
      1) Desquamation of the tips of the fingers and toes is characteristic.
      2) Rash, fever, and lymphadenopathy disappear.
      3) Significant cardiovascular changes, including coronary aneurysm, pericardial effusion, CHF, or myocardial infarction, take place. Approximately 20% of patients manifest coronary artery aneurysm on echo.
      4) Thrombocytosis also occurs during this period, peaking 2 weeks or more after the onset of the illness.
   c. Convalescent phase (until elevated erythrocyte sedimentation rate and platelet count return to normal): deep transverse grooves (Beau lines) may appear across the fingernails and toenails.
2. Echo studies should be obtained to detect coronary artery aneurysm (saccular, fusiform, ectatic) and other reported cardiac dysfunction.
3. The ECG may show reduced QRS voltages, ST-T changes, and prolonged PR interval. Abnormal Q waves (wide and deep) in the limb leads or precordial leads suggest myocardial infarction.
4. CXR film may show cardiomegaly if myocarditis, significant coronary artery abnormality, or valvular regurgitation is present.
5. Abnormal laboratory findings may include the following:
   a. Marked leukocytosis with a shift to the left and elevated acute phase reactants (C-reactive protein α_1-antitrypsin and erythrocyte sedimentation rate) during the acute phase.
   b. Thrombocytosis during the subacute phase (600,000 to more than 1 million/mm^3).
   c. Elevated liver enzymes and mild hyperbilirubinemia.
   d. Elevated myocardial enzymes (such as serum creatine phosphokinase MB fraction) suggest myocardial infarction.
   e. Significantly low levels of HDL cholesterol.

6. Natural history: It is a self-limited disease for most patients. However, coronary aneurysm occurs in 15% to 25% of patients and is responsible for myocardial infarction (fewer than 5%) and mortality (1% to 5%). If the coronary artery remains normal throughout the first month after onset, subsequent development of coronary lesion is extremely unusual. Coronary aneurysm has a tendency to regress within a year in about 50% of patients, but some patients develop stenosis of the coronary artery.

Diagnosis

1. Diagnosis is based on clinical findings. There are no consistently reliable laboratory tests for this disease. Fever and at least four of the remaining five diagnostic criteria are required for the diagnosis (Table 4-2). However, patients with fever and fewer than four criteria can be diagnosed as having Kawasaki disease when coronary artery abnormality is detected.

2. It is necessary to rule out diseases with similar manifestations (measles, group A β-hemolytic streptococcal infection) by appropriate cultures and the use of laboratory tests. Children with Kawasaki disease are extremely irritable (often inconsolable), unlikely to have exudative conjunctivitis, and likely to have a perineal distribution of rash. Other diseases with findings similar to Kawasaki disease such as viral exanthems, sepsis, drug reactions, juvenile rheumatoid arthritis, and Rocky Mountain spotted fever require differentiation.

Treatment: The two goals of therapy are reduction of inflammation within the coronary artery and in the myocardium and prevention of thrombosis by inhibiting platelet aggregation.

1. Single-dose IV γ-globulin 2 g/kg/day with aspirin 80 to 100 mg/kg/day given within 10 days after the onset of illness is the treatment of choice. This significantly reduces the prevalence of short- and long-term coronary artery abnormalities, results in rapid defervescence and resolution of laboratory indices of inflammation, and rapidly resolves the impaired cardiac function.

2. Aspirin is reduced to 3 to 10 mg/kg/day (antiplatelet dose) as a single dose on about day 14 of the illness. Aspirin should be discontinued by 6 to 8 weeks after the onset of illness if no coronary artery abnormalities show up on echo.

3. Serial echo follow-up is important for evaluation of the cardiac status. An echo is indicated as soon as the patient is suspected of having Kawasaki disease. In the absence of giant coronary artery aneurysm, follow-up echoes are indicated 6 to 8 weeks and 6 to 12 months after the onset. If significant abnormalities of the coronary vessels, LV dysfunction, or valvular regurgitation is found, echo should be repeated more often.

4. Occasionally, coronary angiography may be indicated in infants with a very large (giant) aneurysm and in patients with symptoms suggestive of ischemia with positive exercise tests or thallium studies and/or with evidence of myocardial infarction. On rare occasions coronary artery bypass surgery may be indicated.

IV. ACUTE RHEUMATIC FEVER

Etiology: Acute rheumatic fever is a delayed sequela of group A hemolytic streptococcal infection of the pharynx (but not of the skin). It is more common in families with history of rheumatic fever and those of low socioeconomic status. The peak incidence is at 8 years (range 6 to 15 years).

Clinical Manifestations

1. The patient may have had streptococcal pharyngitis 1 to 5 weeks (average 3 weeks) before the onset of symptoms. The latent period may be as long as 2 to 6 months (average 4 months) in cases of isolated chorea.

2. Clinical manifestations of acute rheumatic fever may be grouped into five major criteria, four minor criteria, and supporting evidence of preceding streptococcal infection (Table 4-3).

TABLE 4-3.

Guidelines for the Diagnosis of Initial Attack of Rheumatic Fever
(Jones Criteria, 1992)

Major Manifestations	Minor Manifestations
Carditis Polyarthritis Chorea Erythema marginatum Subcutaneous nodule	**Clinical Findings** Arthralgia Fever **Laboratory Findings** Elevated acute phase reactants (ESR, C-reactive protein) Prolonged PR interval

plus

Supporting Evidence of Antecedent Group A Streptococcal Infection
Positive throat culture or rapid streptococcal antigen test
Elevated or rising streptococcal antibody titer

If supported by evidence of preceding group A streptococcal infection, the presence of two major manifestations or one major and two minor manifestations indicates a high probability of acute rheumatic fever.

From Special Writing Group of the Committee on Rheumatic Fever, Endocarditis, and Kawasaki Disease of the Council of Cardiovascular Disease in the Young, American Heart Association, Circulation 87: 302-307, 1993.

3. Major manifestations
   a. Arthritis is the most common manifestation (60% to 85%), usually involving large joints (knees, ankles, elbows, wrists) with characteristic migratory nature. Arthritis subsides in a few days to weeks even without treatment and does not cause permanent damage.
   b. Carditis affects 40% to 50% of patients. Signs of carditis include some or all of the following:
      1) Tachycardia (out of proportion for the degree of fever).

2) *Significant* heart murmurs (due to MR and/or AR) are almost always present.

3) Pericarditis (friction rub, pericardial effusion, chest pain, and ECG changes).

4) Cardiomegaly on CXR film (caused by pericarditis, pancarditis, or CHF).

5) Signs of CHF (gallop rhythm, distant heart sounds, cardiomegaly). Only carditis can cause permanent cardiac damage. Mild carditis disappears rapidly in weeks, but severe carditis may last for months.

c. Erythema marginatum (10%) with the characteristic nonpruritic serpiginous or annular erythematous rashes is most prominent on the trunk and the inner proximal portions of the extremities.

d. Subcutaneous nodules (2% to 10%) are hard, painless, nonpruritic, freely movable, swelling, 0.2 to 2 cm in diameter. They are usually found symmetrically, singly or in clusters, on the extensor surfaces of both large and small joints, over the scalp, or along the spine.

e. Sydenham chorea, or St. Vitus dance (15%), is found more often in prepubertal girls (8 to 12 years) than in boys. Emotional lability and personality changes are followed by loss of motor coordination, characteristic spontaneous, purposeless movement, and motor weakness. It is often an isolated manifestation; the patient may have no fever, and erythrocyte sedimentation rate (ESR) and antistreptolysin-O (ASO) titers may be normal. Antineuronal antibodies are present in more than 90% of patients. This may be related to dysfunction of basal ganglia and cortical neuronal components.

4. Minor manifestations include fever, arthralgia, elevated acute phase reactants (elevated ESR and CRP) and prolonged PR interval (Table 4-3).

5. Evidence of antecedent group A streptococcal infection

a. History of sore throat or scarlet fever unsubstantiated by laboratory data is not adequate evidence of recent group A streptococcal infection. Positive throat culture or rapid streptococcal antigen test for group A streptococci are less reliable than antibody test because they do not distinguish between recent infection and chronic pharyngeal carriage.

b. Specific antibody tests are the most reliable laboratory evidence of antecedent streptococcal infection capable of producing acute rheumatic fever. An ASO titer above 320 Todd units in children or above 240 Todd units in adults is considered significant. Antideoxyribonuclease B titer of 240 Todd units or more in children or 120 Todd units or more in adults is considered elevated. The Streptozyme test is a relatively simple slide agglutination test but is less standardized and less reproducible than other antibody tests.

Diagnosis: Revised Jones criteria (Table 4-3) consist of three groups of important clinical and laboratory findings that are useful in the diagnosis of acute rheumatic fever. Diagnosis of acute rheumatic fever is highly probable in the presence of either two major manifestations or one major plus two minor manifestations plus evidence of antecedent streptococcal infection. The absence of supporting evidence of a previous group A streptococcal infection makes the diagnosis doubtful.

Management

1. When acute rheumatic fever is suspected, the following lab studies are obtained: CBC, acute phase reactants (ESR, C-reactive protein), throat culture, ASO titer, CXR film and ECG. Cardiology consultation is indicated to clarify any cardiac involvement; 2D echo and Doppler studies are usually performed at that time.

2. Benzathine penicillin G 0.6 million to 1.2 million units is administered IM to eradicate *Streptococcus.* This serves as the first dose of penicillin prophylaxis as well. In patients allergic to penicillin, erythromycin 40 mg/kg/day in two to four doses for 10 days may be substituted for penicillin.

3. Antiinflammatory therapy with salicylates or steroids should not be started until a definite diagnosis is made because it may suppress full development of joint manifestations.

4. It is important to impress on the patient and parents the necessity of preventing subsequent streptococcal infection through continuous antibiotic prophylaxis. The need for SBE prophylaxis for patients with cardiac involvement should also be emphasized.

5. Bed rest is recommended (see Table 4-4). Bed rest is followed by a period of indoor ambulation before the child is allowed to go back to school. The ESR is a helpful guide to the rheumatic activity and therefore to the duration of restricted activities. Full activity is allowed later, when the ESR returns to normal, except for children with significant cardiac involvement.

6. Therapy with antiinflammatory agents should be started as soon as the diagnosis of acute rheumatic fever has been established.

   a. Prednisone 2 mg/kg/day in four divided doses for 2 to 6 weeks is indicated only in cases of severe carditis.

   b. For mild to moderate carditis, aspirin alone is recommended in a dose of 90 to 100 mg/kg/day in four to six divided doses. An adequate blood level of salicylates is 20 to 25 mg/100 ml. This dose is continued for 4 to 8 weeks, depending on the clinical response. Upon improvement the therapy is withdrawn over the following 4 to 6 weeks while acute phase reactants are monitored.

   c. For arthritis aspirin therapy is continued for 2 weeks and gradually withdrawn over the following 2 to 3 weeks. Rapid resolution of joint symptoms with aspirin within 24 to 36 hours is supportive evidence of acute rheumatic fever.

7. Treatment for CHF includes bed rest, oxygen, morphine sulfate, restriction of salt and fluid intake, and furosemide. Digoxin should be used with caution because certain patients with rheumatic carditis are

TABLE 4-4.

General Guide for Bed Rest and Ambulation

	Arthritis Alone	Minimal Carditis	Moderate Carditis	Severe Carditis
Bed rest	1-2 wk	2-3 wk	4-6 wk	2-4 mo
Indoor ambulation	1-2 wk	2-3 wk	4-6 wk	2-3 mo
Outdoor activity (school)	2 wk	2-4 wk	1-3 mo	2-3 mo
Full activity	After 4-6 wk	After 6-10 wk	After 3-6 mo	Variable

Minimal carditis indicates questionable cardiomegaly; moderate carditis indicates definite but mild cardiomegaly; severe carditis indicates marked cardiomegaly or CHF.

supersensitive to digitalis; start with half of the usual recommended dose.

8. Management of Sydenham chorea includes elimination of physical and emotional stress, use of protective measures, and medications such as phenobarbital, chlorpromazine, diazepam, haloperidol, or steroids. Benzathine penicillin G 1.2 million units is given initially for eradication of *Streptococcus* and every 28 days for prevention of recurrence, just as in patients with other rheumatic manifestations. Patients with isolated chorea do not need antiinflammatory agents. Plasma exchange or IV immunoglobulin therapy (because of the presence of antineuronal antibodies) are in the experimental stage.

Prevention

1. Any patient with documented history of rheumatic fever, including those with isolated chorea and those without evidence of rheumatic heart disease, must receive prophylaxis.

2. Ideally, the patient should receive prophylaxis indefinitely. However, many cardiologists recommend discontinuing prophylaxis when the patient is aged 21 to 25 provided the patient does not have evidence of valvular involvement and is not in a high-risk occupation (e.g., schoolteacher, physician, nurse). If the patient has rheumatic valvular disease, the prophylaxis is recommended for a longer (possibly lifelong) period. The chance of recurrence is highest in the first 5 years following the acute rheumatic fever.

3. The method of choice for secondary prevention is benzathine penicillin G, 600,000 units for patients under 60 lbs (27 kg) and 1.2 million units for patients over 60 lbs, given IM every 28 days (not once a month). Although less effective, the following alternative drugs may be used:

   a. Oral penicillin V 125 to 250 mg twice daily.

   b. Oral sulfadiazine 0.5 g once a day for children under 60 lbs and 1 g once a day for children over 60 lbs is equally effective.

   c. If the patient is allergic to penicillin, erythromycin 250 mg twice daily may be used.

4. Primary prevention of rheumatic fever is possible with a 10-day course of penicillin therapy for streptococcal pharyngitis. However, primary prevention does not work for patients who develop subclinical pharyngitis and therefore do not seek medical treatment (30%) or for patients who develop acute rheumatic fever without symptoms of streptococcal pharyngitis (30%).

V. VALVULAR HEART DISEASE

Almost all acquired valvular heart diseases are rheumatic. Mitral valve involvement occurs in about three fourths and aortic valve involvement in about one fourth of all cases with rheumatic heart disease. Stenosis and regurgitation of the same valve usually occur together. Isolated AS of rheumatic origin is extremely rare. Involvement of the tricuspid valve is very rare, and that of the pulmonary valve almost never occurs. Therefore only MS, MR, and AR will be discussed.

A. Mitral Stenosis

Prevalence: Although MS is rare in children (it requires 5 to 10 years from the initial attack), it is the most common valvular involvement in adult rheumatic patients.

Clinical Manifestations

1. Most children with MS are asymptomatic.
2. A narrowly split S2 with accentuated P2 is present if pulmonary hypertension develops. An opening snap followed by a low-frequency middiastolic rumble is audible at the apex. Occasionally a high-frequency diastolic murmur of pulmonary regurgitation (Graham Steell murmur) is present at the ULSB.
3. The ECG may show RAD, RVH, and LAH or CAH. Atrial fibrillation is rare in children.
4. CXR films reveal enlargement of the LA and RV and prominence of the MPA segment. Lung fields may show pulmonary venous congestion, Kerley B lines, and redistribution of PBF to the upper lobes.
5. Echo study is diagnostic. M-mode echo may show large LA dimension, diminished EF slope, and

multiple echoes from thickened mitral leaflets; 2D echo shows a doming of thick mitral leaflets and small mitral valve orifice inscribed by the thickened valve. The Doppler study can estimate the pressure gradient and the level of pulmonary artery pressure.

6. SBE, atrial flutters or fibrillation, and thromboembolism are rare complications in children.

Management

Medical

a. Maintenance of good dental hygiene and SBE prophylaxis if indicated are important. Penicillin or sulfonamide is administered to prevent recurrence of rheumatic fever. Varying degrees of restriction of activity may be indicated.

b. If atrial fibrillation (rare in children) develops, digoxin is used to control ventricular response. If the patient develops pulmonary edema from atrial fibrillation, cardioversion should be attempted. The patient should ideally receive an anticoagulant for 3 to 4 weeks, and quinidine should be started 2 days before the procedure.

c. Balloon valvuloplasty may be tried initially as an alternative to surgical closed commissurotomy; the results are comparable.

Surgical

a. Surgical indications include congestive symptoms (dyspnea on exertion, pulmonary edema, paroxysmal dyspnea), recurrent atrial fibrillation, thromboembolic phenomenon, and hemoptysis.

b. Procedures and mortality

a) Closed mitral commissurotomy remains the procedure of choice for those with a pliable mitral valve without calcification or MR. The operative mortality is less than 1%.

b) Open mitral commissurotomy carries a hospital mortality rate of less than 1% in adults (slightly higher in children).

c) Valve replacement may be indicated in patients with calcified valves and those with MR. Hospital mortality is 2% to 7%. Prosthetic valves (e.g.,

Starr-Edwards, Bjork-Shiley, St. Jude) have the advantage of longer durability but require long-term anticoagulation therapy with its attendant risks (e.g., bleeding, thrombus formation, mechanical malfunction). The bioprostheses (porcine valve, heterograft valve) do not require anticoagulation but tend to deteriorate rapidly in the young.

B. Mitral Regurgitation

Prevalence: MR is the most common valvular involvement in children with rheumatic heart disease.

Clinical Manifestations

1. Children are usually asymptomatic. History of fatigue and palpitation is rarely present.
2. A grade 2 to 4/6 regurgitant systolic murmur is present at the apex and often transmits to the left axilla (best demonstrated on the left decubitus position). A short, low-frequency diastolic flow rumble may be present at the apex. The S2 may split widely (as a result of shortening of LV ejection and early aortic closure). The S3 is commonly present and loud.
3. The ECG is normal in mild MR. LVH or LV dominance is usually present, with occasional LAH in moderate to severe MR.
4. CXR films may show LA and LV enlargement. PVMs are usually normal, but pulmonary venous congestion pattern may appear if CHF develops.
5. 2D echo may show dilated LA and LV. Color mapping and Doppler studies can assess the severity of MR.
6. The patient is relatively stable for a long time, but MS eventually supervenes in some patients. SBE is a rare complication.

Management

Medical

a. SBE prophylaxis if indicated and prophylaxis against recurrence of rheumatic fever are important. Restriction of activity is not indicated in most mild cases.

b. Afterload-reducing agents are useful in maintaining the forward stroke volume. Anticongestive measures (diuretics and digoxin) are indicated if CHF develops. If atrial fibrillation develops (rare in children), digoxin is used to slow the ventricular response.

   Surgical

a. Indications for surgery are not clearly defined, but intractable CHF, progressive cardiomegaly with symptoms, and pulmonary hypertension may be indications.

b. Procedures and mortality: Mitral valve repair surgery is preferred over valve replacement in children as long as the valve is pliable. It carries lower mortality (less than 1%), and anticoagulation is not necessary. Valve replacement is necessary if the valve is thick, scarred, and grossly deformed. Surgical mortality is 2% to 7%. If a prosthetic valve is used, anticoagulation must be maintained.

C. Aortic Regurgitation

Prevalence: AR is less common than MR. Most patients have associated mitral valve disease.

Clinical Manifestations

1. Patients are asymptomatic with mild AR. Exercise tolerance may be reduced with severe AR or CHF.

2. A high-pitched diastolic decrescendo murmur best audible at the 3LICS or 4LICS is present. The longer the murmur, the more severe the regurgitation. A systolic ejection murmur of varying intensity may be present at 2RICS. A middiastolic mitral rumble (Austin-Flint murmur) is occasionally present. Wide pulse pressure and bounding water-hammer pulse develop with severe AR.

3. The ECG is normal or shows LVH.

4. CXR films reveal cardiomegaly involving the LV.

5. 2D echo may show enlargement of the LV. Color flow mapping and Doppler studies can estimate the severity of AR.

6. The patient may remain asymptomatic for a long
   time, but if symptoms begin, many patients deteriorate rapidly. Anginal pain, CHF, and multiple PVCs
   are unfavorable signs.

Management

Medical

a. SBE prophylaxis on indications and prophylaxis
   against recurrence of rheumatic fever are important. Restriction of activity is not needed for mild
   cases, but varying degrees of restriction are indicated in more severe cases.

b. If CHF develops, digoxin, diuretics, and afterload-
   reducing agents may be beneficial, but benefits are
   rarely maintained.

Surgical

a. Indications: A major clinical decision in AR is
   the timing of aortic valve replacement. Ideally, it
   should be performed before irreversible dilatation
   of the LV develops, but there is no reliable method
   of determining that point. The following findings
   have been used as indications for the valve replacement therapy. (1) Symptoms such as anginal pain
   or dyspnea on exertion. (2) Even in asymptomatic patients, significant cardiomegaly (with the CT
   ratio above 55%), ejection fraction less than 40%,
   or stress test–induced symptoms.

b. Procedure and mortality: Aortic valve replacement under cardiopulmonary bypass carries
   mortality of about 2% to 5%. The antibiotic-
   sterilized aortic homograft has been widely used
   and appears to be the device of choice. The porcine heterograft has the risk of accelerated degeneration. The Bjork-Shiley and the St. Jude
   prostheses require anticoagulation and are not
   well suited to young patients. Pulmonary-root
   autograft (Ross procedure) may be an attractive
   alternative (Fig 4-2) in selected adolescents and
   young adults. In this procedure the patient's own
   pulmonary valve and the adjacent pulmonary
   artery replace the diseased aortic valve and the

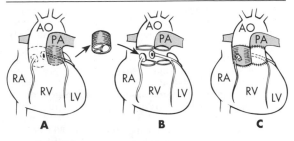

FIG. 4-2.
Ross procedure (pulmonary root autograft). **A,** Two horizontal lines on the aorta and two broken circles around the coronary artery ostia are lines of proposed incision. The pulmonary valve with a small rim of RV muscle and the adjacent PA are removed. **B,** The aortic valve and the adjacent aorta have been removed, leaving buttons of aortic tissue around the coronary arteries. **C,** The pulmonary autograft is sutured to the aortic annulus and to the distal aorta, and the coronary arteries are sutured to openings made in the PA. The pulmonary valve is replaced with either an aortic or pulmonary allograft.

adjacent aorta. The coronary arteries are detached from the aorta and implanted into the pulmonary artery. A bioprosthetic valve is placed in the pulmonary valve position. Surgical mortality is near zero. This procedure does not necessitate anticoagulant therapy, and the autograft may last longer than porcine bioprosthesis.

D. Mitral Valve Prolapse

Prevalence: MVP may occur in up to 5% of children. It is more common in adults, with female preponderance (2:1).

Pathology and Cause

1. Thick and redundant mitral valve leaflets due to myxomatous degeneration bulge into the mitral annulus. The posterior leaflet is more commonly and more severely affected than the anterior leaflet.

2. It is idiopathic in more than 50% of cases. It is familial in the primary form (with autosomal dominant inheritance). CHD is present in 30% of cases, with ASD the most common defect. Nearly all patients with Marfan syndrome have MVP. MVP may be seen with other connective tissue disorders.

Clinical Manifestations

1. Although MVP is usually asymptomatic, history of nonexertional chest pain, palpitation, and rarely syncope may be elicited.

2. An asthenic build with a high incidence (80%) of thoracic skeletal anomalies (e.g., pectus excavatum, straight back, and scoliosis) is common. The midsystolic click with or without a late systolic murmur at the apex is the hallmark of this condition. The presence or absence of the click and murmur, as well as their timing, are variable from one examination to the next.

   a. The click and murmur may be brought out by held expiration, left decubitus position, sitting, standing, or leaning forward. They may disappear on inspiration.

   b. Various maneuvers can alter the timing of the click and the murmur. The click moves toward the S1 and the murmur lengthens by maneuvers that decrease the LV volume (e.g., standing, sitting, Valsalva strain phase, tachycardia, administration of amyl nitrite). The click moves toward the S2, and the murmur shortens by maneuvers that increase the LV volume (e.g., squatting, hand grip exercise, Valsalva release phase, bradycardia, administration of pressor agents or propranolol).

3. The ECG shows flat or inverted T waves in II, III, and aVF (20% to 60%). Arrhythmias (SVT, PACs, and PVCs) and conduction disturbances (first degree AV block, WPW syndrome, prolonged QT interval, or RBBB) are occasionally present.

4. CXR films are usually normal except for LA enlargement in patients with severe MR.

5. 2D echo findings of a superior displacement of the mitral valve leaflet in the parasternal long axis view

is diagnostic. The superior displacement seen only on the apical four-chamber view is not diagnostic, since more than 30% of preselected normal children show this finding: the saddle-shaped mitral valve ring explains this finding. The mitral valve leaflets are often thick, and MR is occasionally demonstrable. Many children with a midsystolic click (usually without late systolic murmur) fail to show the diagnostic sign of MVP by 2D echo studies, although thickened leaflets and the bowing of the leaflets within the LV cavity are frequently found. This finding may be explained by the fact that MVP is a progressive disease with a less than full manifestation in children.

6. The majority of patients are asymptomatic, particularly during childhood. Complications are rare during childhood, but those reported in adult patients include sudden death from ventricular arrhythmias, SBE, spontaneous rupture of chordae tendineae, progressive MR, CHF, and arrhythmias and conduction disturbances.

Management

1. Asymptomatic patients require no treatment or restriction of activity. SBE prophylaxis is observed if indicated.

2. Patients who are symptomatic (palpitations, light-headedness, dizziness, or syncope) or who have arrhythmias should undergo ambulatory ECG monitoring and/or treadmill exercise testing. Propranolol or another β-adrenergic blocker is the drug of choice for arrhythmias and chest pain. Another drug, such as calcium blockers, quinidine, or procainamide, may be effective in some patients.

3. Reconstructive surgery or mitral valve replacement may be indicated in rare patients with severe MR.

VI. CARDIAC TUMORS

Prevalence: Cardiac tumors are extremely rare among children.

Pathology: The most common cardiac tumor among children is rhabdomyoma. In infants less than 1 year old, more than 75% of tumors are rhabdomyomas and teratomas, and in children ages 1 to 15, 80% of cardiac tumors are rhabdomyomas, fibromas, and myxomas. More than 90% of primary tumors are benign. Myxomas are extremely rare in children, although the LA myxoma is the most common type of cardiac tumor in adults. Myxomas can produce hemodynamic disturbances by interfering with mitral valve function or cause thromboembolic phenomena in the systemic circulation. Surgical removal is usually successful.

Clinical Manifestations

1. Syncope or chest pain may be a presenting complaint. Rarely, postural variations in symptoms are present with pedunculated tumors.

2. Clinical manifestations of cardiac tumors are often nonspecific, and they vary primarily with the location of the tumor. Tumors near cardiac valves may produce heart murmurs of stenosis or regurgitation of the valves. Tumors involving the conduction tissue may manifest with arrhythmias or conduction disturbances. Intracavitary tumors may produce inflow or outflow obstruction or thromoembolic phenomena. Invasion of the myocardium by the tumor (mural tumors) may result in heart failure or cardiac arrhythmias. Pericardial tumors, which may signal malignancy, may produce pericardial effusion and cardiac tamponade or features simulating infective pericarditis. Occasionally, for unknown reasons, fever and general malaise may manifest, especially with myxomas.

3. The ECG may show nonspecific ST-T changes, an infarct-like pattern, low-voltage QRS complexes, preexcitation, arrhythmias, or conduction disturbances.

4. CXR film may occasionally reveal altered contour of the heart with or without changes in pulmonary vascular markings.

5. Echo and Doppler studies are diagnostic and can determine hemodynamic significance of the lesion. Cardiac tumors are often found on a routine echo study without suspicion of the diagnosis, especially in newborns and small infants.

   a. Multiple intraventricular tumors are most likely rhabdomyomas in infants and children.
   b. A solitary tumor of varying size arising from the ventricular septum or the ventricular wall is likely to be fibroma.
   c. Left atrial tumors, especially when pedunculated, are usually myxomas.
   d. An intrapericardial tumor arising near the great arteries is most likely a teratoma.
   e. Pericardial effusion suggests a possibility of a secondary malignant tumor.

   Treatment: Surgery is indicated for symptoms of cardiac failure or ventricular arrhythmias refractory to medical treatment and for inlet or outlet obstruction.

1. A successful complete resection of a fibroma is possible.
2. In asymptomatic patients with multiple rhabdomyomas, surgery should be delayed because of the possibility of spontaneous regression of the tumor.
3. Surgical removal, a standard procedure for myxomas, generally has a a favorable outcome.
4. If there is an extensive myocardial involvement, surgical treatment is not possible. Cardiac transplantation may be an option in such cases.

ARRHYTHMIAS AND ATRIOVENTRICULAR CONDUCTION DISTURBANCES

V

Normal heart rate varies with age: the younger the child, the faster the heart rate. Therefore, the definitions used for adults of bradycardia (fewer than 60 beats/min) and tachycardia (above 100 beats/min) have little significance for children. A child has tachycardia when the heart rate is beyond the upper limit of normal for age, and bradycardia, when the heart rate is slower than the lower limit of normal (see Table 1-12).

I. BASIC ARRHYTHMIAS

A. Rhythms Originating in the Sinus Node

All rhythms that originate in the sinoatrial (SA) node (sinus rhythm) have two important characteristics. Five rhythms (Fig 5-1) all show these characteristics.

    a. A P wave is present in front of each QRS complex with a regular PR interval. (The PR interval may be prolonged, as in first degree AV block).

    b. The P axis is between 0 and +90 degrees, (producing upright P waves in lead II and inverted P waves in aVR) (see Fig 1-12).

Regular Sinus Rhythm: The rhythm is regular and the rate is normal for age. The two characteristics of sinus rhythm are present. This is normal rhythm at any age.

Sinus Tachycardia

    Description: The characteristics of sinus rhythm are present. A rate above 140 beats/min in children and

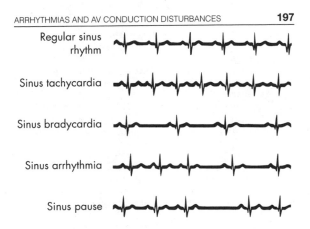

FIG. 5-1.
Normal and abnormal rhythms originating in the sinus node. (From Park MK, Guntheroth WG: *How to Read Pediatric ECGs,* ed. 3. St. Louis, Mosby, 1992.)

above 160 beats/min in infants may be significant. The heart rate is usually lower than 200 beats/min in sinus tachycardia.

Causes: Anxiety, fever, hypovolemia, circulatory shock, anemia, CHF, catecholamines, thyrotoxicosis, and myocardial disease are possible causes.

Significance: Increased cardiac work is well tolerated by the healthy myocardium.

Treatment: The underlying cause is treated.

Sinus Bradycardia

Description: The characteristics of sinus rhythm are present. A rate below 80 beats/min in newborn infants and below 60 beats/min in older children may be significant.

Causes: Sinus bradycardia may occur in trained athletes. Vagal stimulation, increased intracranial pressure, hypothyroidism, hypothermia, hypoxia, hy-

perkalemia, and drugs such as digitalis and
β-adrenergic blockers are possible causes.

Significance: Some patients with marked bradycar-
dias do not maintain normal cardiac output.

Treatment: The underlying cause is treated.

Sinus Arrhythmia

Description: There is a phasic variation in the heart
rate, increasing during inspiration and decreasing
during expiration, and the two characteristics of
sinus rhythm are maintained.

Causes: This normal phenomenon is due to a phasic
variation in the firing rate of cardiac autonomic
nerves with the phase of respiration.

Significance: There is no hemodynamic significance.

Treatment: No treatment is indicated.

Sinus Pause

Description: In *sinus pause* there is a momentary ces-
sation of sinus node pacemaker activity resulting in
the absence of P wave and QRS complex for a
relatively short duration. *Sinus arrest* lasts longer
and usually results in an escape beat (such as nodal
escape).

Causes: Increased vagal tone, hypoxia, digitalis toxicity, and sick sinus syndrome.

Significance: No hemodynamic significance is
present.

Treatment: Treatment is rarely indicated except in
sick sinus syndrome and digitalis toxicity.

Sick Sinus Syndrome

Description: The sinus node fails to function as the
dominant pacemaker of the heart or performs
abnormally slowly, producing a variety of arrhythmias. The arrhythmias may include profound
sinus bradycardia, sinus arrest with junctional escape, ectopic atrial or nodal rhythm, SVT, and
bradytachy-arrhythmia.

Causes: Extensive cardiac surgery involving the atria
(e.g., the Mustard or Senning procedure or the
Fontan operation), arteritis or focal myocarditis,
and occasionally idiopathic involving an otherwise
normal heart.

Significance: Bradytachyarrhythmia is the most worrisome rhythm. Profound bradycardia following a period of tachycardia (overdrive suppression) can cause syncope and even death.

Treatment: An antiarrhythmic drug, such as propranolol or quinidine, to suppress tachycardia is indicated. Demand ventricular pacemaker may be required for symptomatic patients with episodes of extreme bradycardia.

B. Rhythms Originating in the Atrium

Atrial arrhythmias (Fig 5-2) are characterized by the following:

    a. P waves of unusual contour (abnormal P axis), and/or an abnormal number of P waves per QRS complex.

    b. QRS complexes of normal duration (but with occasional wide QRS duration caused by aberrancy).

Premature Atrial Contraction

Description: In PAC the QRS complex occurs prematurely with abnormal P wave morphology. There is an incomplete compensatory pause; i.e., the length of two cycles including one premature beat is less than the length of two normal cycles. Occasionally, PACs are not followed by the QRS complex (nonconducted PAC).

Causes: Follows cardiac surgery and digitalis toxicity; also appears in healthy children, including the newborn.

Significance: There is no hemodynamic significance.

Treatment: Usually no treatment is indicated except in digitalis toxicity.

Wandering Atrial Pacemaker

Description: Gradual changes in the shape of P waves and PR intervals occur. The QRS complex is normal.

Causes: This is seen in otherwise healthy children.

Significance: There is no clinical significance.

Treatment: No treatment is indicated.

Atrial Tachycardia: Atrial tachycardia is difficult to separate from the rarer nodal tachycardia or AV

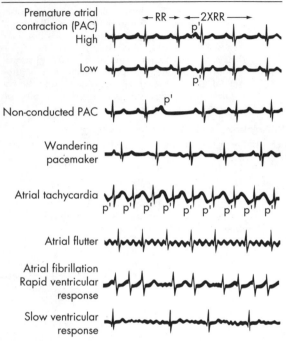

FIG. 5-2.
Arrhythmias originating in the atrium. (From Park MK, Guntheroth WG: *How to Read Pediatric ECGs,* ed 3. St. Louis, Mosby, 1992.)

reentrant tachycardia. This has led to the use of the term *supraventricular tachycardia* (SVT) to include both atrial and nodal tachycardias. Therefore, atrial tachycardia will be discussed later, in the section on supraventricular tachycardia.

Atrial Flutter

Description: Atrial flutter is characterized by a fast atrial rate (F waves with saw-tooth configuration) of about 300 beats/min, the ventricle responding with varying degrees of block (e.g., 2:1, 3:1, 4:1), and normal QRS complexes (Fig 5-2).

Causes: Structural heart disease with dilated atria, myocarditis, previous surgery involving atria (Mustard procedure or ASD repair), and digitalis toxicity.

Significance: The ventricular rate determines the eventual cardiac output; a too-rapid ventricular rate may decrease the cardiac output.

Treatment: Digitalization if the arrhythmia is not the result of digitalis toxicity. Digitalis increases the AV block and slows the ventricular rate. Propranolol may be added. Electric cardioversion may be required. Digitalis should be discontinued for at least 48 hours prior to cardioversion. Warfarin (Coumadin) is recommended before cardioversion to prevent embolization. Rapid atrial pacing with a catheter in the esophagus or the RA can be effective when cardioversion is contraindicated (e.g., in digitalized patients). Quinidine may prevent recurrence.

Atrial Fibrillation

Description: Atrial fibrillation is characterized by an extremely fast atrial rate (f wave at 350 to 600 beats/min) and an irregularly irregular ventricular response with normal QRS complexes (Fig 5-2).

Causes: Same as those for atrial flutter.

Significance: Atrial fibrillation usually suggests a significant pathology. Rapid ventricular rate and the loss of coordinated contraction of the atria and ventricles decrease cardiac output. Atrial thrombus formation is quite common.

Treatment: Digoxin is given to slow the ventricular rate. Propranolol may be added if necessary. Cardioversion may be indicated, but recurrence is common. Patients should be anticoagulated for 3 to 4 weeks before and after the cardioversion to prevent embolization of atrial thrombus. Quinidine is used to prevent recurrence.

Supraventricular Tachycardia

    Description: Three groups of tachycardia are included in SVT: atrial (ectopic or nonreciprocating), nodal (or AV junctional), and AV reentrant (or reciprocating). The great majority of SVTs are due to reentry AV tachycardia rather than rapid firing of a single focus in the atria (atrial tachycardia) or in the AV node (nodal tachycardia).

    The heart rate is extremely rapid and regular (usually 240 plus or minus 40 beats/min). The P wave is usually invisible, but when it is visible, it has an abnormal P axis and either precedes or follows the QRS complex. The QRS duration is usually normal, but occasionally aberrancy will prolong the QRS, making differentiation of this arrhythmia from ventricular tachycardia difficult.

a. *AV reentrant tachycardia* is the most common tachyarrhythmia seen among the children. It used to be called paroxysmal atrial tachycardia because its onset and termination were characteristically abrupt. In SVT due to reentry two pathways are involved, at least one of which is the AV node and the other is an accessory pathway. The accessory pathway may be an anatomically separate bypass tract such as the bundle of Kent (which produces *accessory reciprocating AV tachycardia*) or only functionally separate, as in a dual AV node pathway (which produces *nodal reciprocating AV tachycardia*). Patients with the bundle of Kent frequently have preexcitation (or WPW) syndrome.

b. *Ectopic, or nonreciprocating, atrial tachycardia* is a rare mechanism of SVT in which rapid firing of a single focus in the atrium is responsible for the tachycardia. In contrast to reciprocating atrial tachycardia, in ectopic atrial tachycardia the heart rate varies substantially during the course of a day, and second-degree AV block may develop.

c. *Nodal tachycardia* may superficially resemble atrial tachycardia because the P wave is buried in the T waves of the preceding beat and becomes invisible in the latter, but the rate of nodal tachycardia is relatively slower (120 to 200 beats/min) than the rate of atrial tachycardia.

Causes: No demonstrable heart disease (idiopathic) is present in about half of the patients; idiopathy is more common in young infants than in older children. WPW syndrome, present in 10% to 20% of patients, is evident only after conversion to sinus rhythm. Some congenital heart defects (e.g., Ebstein's anomaly, single ventricle, L-TGA) are more prone to this arrhythmia.

Significance: It may decrease cardiac output and result in CHF (with irritability, tachypnea, poor feeding, and pallor). When CHF develops, the infant's condition can deteriorate rapidly.

Treatment

a. Vagal stimulatory maneuvers (e.g., carotid sinus massage, gagging, pressure on an eyeball) may be effective in older children, but they are rarely effective in infants.

b. Placing an icebag on the face (up to 10 seconds) is often successful in infants.

c. Adenosine has negative chronotropic, dromotropic, and inotropic actions of very short duration (a half-life of less than 1.5 sec) with minimal hemodynamic consequences. It transiently blocks the AV conduction and sinus node pacemaking activity. Adenosine may be the drug of choice in the treatment of SVT, as it terminates almost all SVT in which the AV node forms part of the reentry circuit. It is not effective for nonreciprocating atrial tachycardia, atrial flutter or fibrillation, or ventricular tachycardia. Adenosine also has differential diagnostic utility for both narrow- and wide-complex *regular* tachycardia (but is not recommended for the management of irregular tachycardias). Its transient AV block may unmask atrial activities by slowing the ventricular rate and help in clarifying the mechanism of certain supraventricular arrhythmias. It is given in rapid IV bolus followed by a saline flush, starting at 50 µg/kg and increasing in increments of 50 µg/kg every 1 to 2 min (max 250 µg/kg). The usual effective dose in children is 100 to 150 µg/kg. Digitalization follows in small children to prevent recurrence of the tachycardia.

d. If adenosine is not available, initial cardioversion may be performed in infants with CHF, because cardioversion carries a risk of inducing ventricular tachycardia in digitalized patients. The initial dose of 0.5 joules/kg may be increased step by step up to 2 joules/kg. This is followed by digitalization.

e. Digitalization may be used in infants without CHF and those with mild CHF.

f. If the patient is not in CHF, adenosine is not available, and digitalis is not effective, IV infusion of phenylephrine may be tried when a rapid conversion to sinus rhythm is desirable. It raises blood pressure abruptly and converts the tachycardia by reflex increase in vagal tone. This method is not recommended in infants with CHF.

g. Intravenous administration of propranolol or verapamil may be tried, but these drugs may produce extreme bradycardia and hypotension in infants less than age 1 (and should be avoided when possible). When the decision is made to administer these drugs, they should be given step-by-step in small doses with careful monitoring of vital signs and with readiness to respond to adverse effects.

h. Overdrive suppression by transesophageal pacing in the intensive care unit or by atrial pacing in the cardiac catheterization lab may be indicated for children already taking digitalis.

i. Prevention of recurrence of SVT with maintenance dose of digoxin for 3 to 6 months is recommended. In children over age 8 with WPW syndrome, propranolol or atenolol is preferable to digoxin.

j. In occasional patients with WPW syndrome, catheter ablation or surgical interruption of accessory

pathways should be considered if medical management fails.

C. Rhythms Originating in the AV Node

Rhythms originating in the AV node (Fig 5-3) are characterized by the following:

a. The P wave may be absent, or inverted P waves may
follow the QRS complex.
b. The QRS complex is usually normal in duration
and configuration.

Nodal Premature Beats

Description: A normal QRS complex occurs prematurely. P waves are usually absent, but inverted P
waves may follow QRS complexes. The compensatory pause may be complete or incomplete.

Causes: Usually idiopathic in an otherwise normal
heart but may result from cardiac surgery or digitalis toxicity.

Significance: Usually no hemodynamic significance.

Treatment: Treatment is not indicated unless caused
by digitalis toxicity.

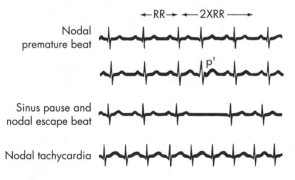

FIG. 5-3.
Arrhythmias originating in the AV node. (From Park MK, Guntheroth
WG: *How to Read Pediatric ECGs,* ed 3. St. Louis, Mosby, 1992.)

Nodal Escape Beat

Description: When the sinus node impulse fails to reach the AV node, the node-His (NH) region of the AV node will initiate an impulse (nodal or junctional escape beat). The QRS complex occurs later than the anticipated normal beat. The P wave may be absent, or an inverted P wave may follow the QRS complex (Fig 5-3).

Causes: It may follow cardiac surgery involving the atria (the Mustard or Senning procedure) or may be seen in otherwise healthy children.

Significance: Little hemodynamic significance.

Treatment: Generally no specific treatment is required.

Nodal or Junctional Rhythm

Description: If there is a persistent failure of the sinus node, the AV node may function as the main pacemaker of the heart with a relatively slow rate (40 to 60 beats/min). Either there are no P waves or inverted P waves follow QRS complexes.

Causes: It may be seen in an otherwise normal heart, after cardiac surgery, in conditions of an increased vagal tone (e.g., increased intracranial pressure, pharyngeal stimulation), and with digitalis toxicity.

Significance: The slow heart rate may significantly decrease the cardiac output and produce symptoms.

Treatment: No treatment is indicated if the patient is asymptomatic. Atropine or electric pacing is indicated for symptoms. Treatment is directed to digitalis toxicity if caused by digitalis.

Accelerated Nodal Rhythm

Description: In the presence of normal sinus rate and AV conduction, if the AV node (NH region) with enhanced automaticity captures the pacemaker function (60 to 120 beats/min), the rhythm is called accelerated nodal (or AV junctional). Either P waves are absent or inverted P waves follow QRS complexes.

Causes: Idiopathic, digitalis toxicity, myocarditis, or cardiac surgery.

Significance: Little hemodynamic significance.

Treatment: No treatment is necessary unless caused by digitalis toxicity.

Nodal Tachycardia

Description: The ventricular rate varies from 120 to 200 beats/min. The QRS complex is usually normal, but aberration may occur. Nodal tachycardia is difficult to separate from atrial tachycardia. Therefore, both arrhythmias are grouped as SVT.

Causes: Similar to those of atrial tachycardia.

Significance: Too fast a rate may decrease the cardiac output.

Treatment: Treatment is not indicated if the rate is slower than 130 beats/min. Although digoxin is the drug of choice for most cases of atrial SVT, it may be contraindicated in the true form of nodal tachycardia. In that case quinidine is probably the drug of choice.

D. Rhythms Originating in the Ventricle

Ventricular arrhythmias (Fig 5-4) are characterized by the following:

   a. Bizarre and wide QRS complexes with T waves pointing in the opposite directions.

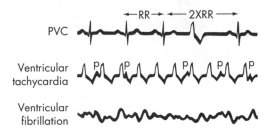

FIG. 5-4.
Ventricular arrhythmias. (From Park MK, Guntheroth WG: *How to Read Pediatric ECGs,* ed 3. St. Louis, Mosby, 1992.)

b. QRS complexes randomly related to P waves, if visible.

Premature Ventricular Contraction

Description

a. In PVC a bizarre, wide QRS complex comes earlier than anticipated, with the T wave pointing in the opposite direction. There is usually a full compensatory pause (i.e., the length of two cycles, including the premature beat, is the same as that of two normal cycles).

b. PVCs may be classified into several types.

1) By interrelationship of PVCs

a) Ventricular *bigeminy* or *coupling:* each abnormal QRS complex alternates with normal QRS complex regularly.

b) Ventricular *trigeminy:* each abnormal QRS complex follows two normal QRS complexes regularly.

c) *Couplets:* Two abnormal QRS complexes come in sequence.

d) *Triplets:* Three abnormal QRS complexes come in sequence. Three or more successive PVCs arbitrarily are termed ventricular tachycardia.

2) By similarity among abnormal QRS complexes

a) Uniform, or unifocal, PVCs: Abnormal QRS complexes have the same configuration in a single lead. It is assumed that they originate from a single focus.

b) Multiform, or multifocal, PVCs: Abnormal QRS complexes have different configurations in a single lead. It is assumed that they originate from different foci.

Causes: PVCs may be seen in otherwise healthy children. Left ventricular false tendon, myocarditis, myocardial injury or infarction, cardiomyopathy (dilated or hypertrophic), cardiac tumors, right ventricular dysplasia (RV cardiomyopathy), long QT syndrome, preoperative or postoperative congenital or acquired heart disease, digitalis toxicity, certain drugs (such as catecholamines, theophylline, caffeine, amphetamines, and some anesthetic agents) and MVP are also possible causes.

Significance

a. Occasional PVCs are benign in children, particularly if they are uniform and disappear or decrease in frequency with exercise.

b. PVCs are more likely to be significant if (1) they are associated with underlying heart disease (e.g., preoperative or postoperative status, MVP, cardiomyopathy), (2) there is a history of syncope or a family history of sudden death, (3) they are precipitated by or increase in frequency with activity, (4) they are multiform, particularly couplets, (5) there are runs of PVC with symptoms, or (6) there are incessant or frequent episodes of paroxysmal ventricular tachycardia.

Investigation for PVCs

a. In children with an otherwise normal heart, occasional isolated uniform PVCs that are suppressed by exercise probably do not require extensive investigations.

b. Children with frequent uniform PVCs including ventricular bigeminy and trigeminy need not be treated or followed by a cardiologist if the ECG, the echocardiogram, and the exercise test results are normal. The ECG is obtained to detect ST-T changes and QTc prolongation. Echo studies will detect structural heart disease, including hypertrophic cardiomyopathy, MVP and RV dysplasia, as well as LV false tendon. The stress test may induce or exacerbate arrhythmias (which indicates an underlying heart disease) and may reveal prolonged QTc during the recovery period.

c. Children with multiform PVCs and ventricular couplets should have 24-hour Holter monitoring, even if they have a structurally normal heart by these tests, to detect the severity and extent of ventricular arrhythmias. They should be evaluated annually with echo, stress test, and 24-hour Holter monitoring.

d. Patients with symptomatic ventricular arrhythmias

or sustained ventricular tachycardia and a seem-
ingly normal heart should undergo cardiac catheterization (which is better than echo for the diagnosis of right ventricular dysplasia). Occasionally
invasive electrophysiologic studies and RV endomyocardial biopsy may be indicated.

Treatment

a. PVCs that cause no symptoms and have no hemodynamic consequences in patients with normal
heart do not require treatment.

b. All children with symptomatic ventricular arrhythmias should be treated.

1) Frequent PVCs may require treatment with an
IV bolus of lidocaine 1 mg/kg/dose followed
by an IV drip of lidocaine 20 to 50 µg/kg/min.

2) β-Blockers (such as atenolol 1 to 2 mg/kg PO in
a single daily dose) are effective for cardiomyopathy and occasionally for right ventricular
dysplasia.

3) Other antiarrhythmic drugs such as diphenylhydantoin (Dilantin) or mexiletine may prove to
be effective. Avoid antiarrhythmic agents that
prolong the QT interval such as class IA
(quinidine, procainamide), class IC (encainide, flecainide), and class III (amiodarone,
bretylium).

Ventricular Tachycardia

Description: VT is a series of three or more PVCs with
a heart rate of 120 to 200 beats/min. QRS complexes are wide and bizarre, with T waves pointing
in opposite directions. QRS contours during the VT
may be unchanging (uniform, monophasic), or
may vary randomly (multiform, polymorphous, or
pleomorphic). Torsade de pointes (meaning "twist-
ing of the points") is a distinct form of polymorphic
VT characterized by a paroxysm of VT during which
there are progressive changes in the amplitude and
polarity of QRS complexes separated by a narrow
transition QRS complex. They occur in patients
with marked QT prolongation. VT is sometimes

difficult to differentiate from SVT with aberrant conduction. However, wide QRS tachycardia in an infant or child must be considered VT until proven otherwise.

Causes: Similar to those listed for PVCs except for normal children. Torsade de pointes may be caused by drugs or chemicals that prolong the QT interval, such as antiarrhythmic drugs, especially class IA (quinidine, procainamide), class IC (encainide, flecainide), and class III (amiodarone, bretylium), phenothiazines (Thorazine, Mellaril), tricyclic antidepressants (imipramine, desipra mine), certain antibiotics (ampicillin, erythromycin, trimethoprim-sulfamethoxazole) the antihistamine terfenadine (Seldane), and organophosphate insecticides.

Significance: Usually signifies a serious myocardial pathology or dysfunction. Cardiac output may decrease notably and may deteriorate to ventricular fibrillation.

Treatment

a. Prompt synchronized cardioversion (0.5 to 1.0 joules/kg) if the patient is unconscious or if there is evidence of low cardiac output.

b. If the patient is conscious, an IV bolus of lidocaine 1 mg/kg over 1 to 2 min followed by an IV drip of lidocaine 20 to 50 µg/kg/min may be effective.

c. If lidocaine is unsuccessful, bretylium tosylate 5 mg/kg IV over 8 to 10 min may be tried.

d. An IV bolus injection of magnesium sulfate 2 g has recently been reported to be very effective and safe for torsade de pointes in adult patients. The conventional treatment for torsade de pointes is aimed at shortening the QT interval by increasing heart rate (through isoproterenol infusion or cardiac pacing).

e. A search for reversible conditions contributing to the initiation and maintenance of VT should be made and the conditions (such as hypokalemia, hypoxemia) corrected if possible.

f. Recurrence may be prevented with administration

of propranolol, atenolol, diphenylhydantoin, or
quinidine.
g. If antiarrhythmic control is inadequate, invasive
electrophysiologic studies should be considered.
h. Rarely, ventricular or atrial pacing combined with
antiarrhythmic agents, implantable cardioverter or
defibrillator, surgical excision, or ablation techniques may be tested in selected patients.

Aberration: When a supraventricular impulse prematurely reaches the AV node or bundle of His, it may
find one bundle branch excitable and the other still
refractory. Therefore, the resulting QRS complex
resembles a bundle branch block pattern. The right
bundle branch usually has a longer refractory period
than the left, producing QRS complexes similar to
those of RBBB. The following features are helpful in
differentiating aberrant ventricular conduction from
ectopic ventricular impulses:

1. An rsR' pattern in V1, resembling QRS complexes
   of RBBB, suggests aberration. In a ventricular
   ectopic beat the QRS morphology is bizarre and
   does not resemble the classic form of RBBB or
   LBBB.
2. Occasional wide QRS complexes following P waves
   with regular PR intervals suggest an aberration.
3. The presence of a ventricular fusion complex is a
   reliable sign of ventricular ectopic rhythm.

Ventricular Fibrillation

Description: Ventricular fibrillation is characterized
by bizarre QRS complexes of varying sizes and
configuration. The rate is rapid and irregular.

Causes: Postoperative state, severe hypoxia, hyperkalemia, digitalis or quinidine toxicity, myocarditis,
myocardial infarction, and drugs (catecholamines,
anesthetics, etc) are possible causes.

Significance: It is usually fatal, since it results in
ineffective circulation.

Treatment: Immediate CPR, including electric
defibrillation at 2 joules/kg, is required.

II. DISTURBANCES OF ATRIOVENTRICULAR CONDUCTION

AV block is a disturbance in conduction between the normal sinus impulse and the eventual ventricular response. It is classified according to the severity of the conduction disturbance as first degree, second degree, or third degree (Fig 5-5).

A. First-degree AV Block

Description: There is a prolongation of the PR interval beyond the upper limits of normal (see Table 1-14) due to an abnormal delay in conduction through the AV node (Fig 5-5).

Causes: Some healthy children, acute rheumatic fever, cardiomyopathies, CHDs (e.g., ASD, Ebstein anomaly, ECD), cardiac surgery, and digitalis toxicity.

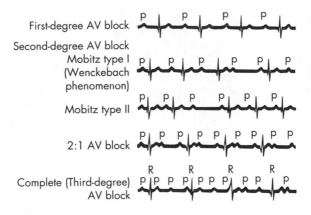

FIG. 5-5.
Atrioventricular block. (From Park MK, Guntheroth WG: *How to Read Pediatric ECGs,* ed 3. St. Louis, Mosby, 1992.)

Significance: Usually no hemodynamic disturbance results. Sometimes it may progress to a more advanced AV block.

Treatment: No treatment is indicated except in digitalis toxicity.

B. Second-degree AV Block

Some but not all P waves are followed by QRS complexes (dropped beats). There are several types:

Mobitz Type I (Wenckebach Phenomenon)

Description: The PR interval becomes progressively prolonged until one QRS complex is dropped completely (Fig 5-5).

Causes: Myocarditis, cardiomyopathy, myocardial infarction, CHD, cardiac surgery, and digitalis toxicity; it also affects otherwise healthy children.

Significance: The block is at the level of the AV node. It usually does not progress to complete heart block.

Treatment: The underlying cause is treated.

Mobitz Type II

Description: The AV conduction is all or none: there is either normal AV conduction or the conduction is completely blocked (Fig 5-5).

Causes: Same as for Mobitz type I.

Significance: The block is at the level of the bundle of His. It is more serious than type I block, since it may progress to complete heart block.

Treatment: The underlying cause is treated. Prophylactic pacemaker therapy may be indicated.

Two-to-one (or Higher) AV Block

Description: A QRS complex follows every second (third or fourth) P wave resulting in 2:1 (3:1 or 4:1, respectively) AV block (Fig 5-5).

Causes: Similar to other second-degree AV blocks.

Significance: The block is usually at the AV nodal level and occasionally at the level of the bundle of His. It may occasionally progress to complete heart block.

Treatment: The underlying cause is treated. Electrophysiologic studies may be necessary to determine the level of the block. Occasional pacemaker therapy.

C. Third-degree AV Block (Complete Heart Block)

Description: In third-degree AV block the atrial and ventricular activities are entirely independent of each other (Fig 5-5): The P waves are regular (with regular PP interval) with a rate comparable to the heart rate of the patient's age. The QRS complexes are also quite regular (with regular RR interval) with a rate much slower than the P rate.

In *congenital* complete heart block, the duration of the QRS complex is normal, since the pacemaker for the QRS complex is at a level higher than the bifurcation of the bundle of His. The ventricular rate is faster (50 to 80 beats/min) than in the acquired type. In surgically induced or *acquired* (post–myocardial infarction) complete heart block, the QRS duration is prolonged, and the ventricular rate is in the range of 40 to 50 beats/min. The pacemaker for the QRS complex is at a level below the bifurcation of the bundle of His.

Causes

a. The congenital type may be an isolated anomaly (without associated CHD). Maternal lupus erythematosus or mixed connective tissue disease or CHD such as L-TGA may be the cause of complete heart block.

b. The acquired type is usually a complication of cardiac surgery in children. Rarely severe myocarditis, acute rheumatic fever, mumps, diphtheria, cardiomyopathies, tumors in the conduction system, or overdose of certain drugs causes it. It may also follow myocardial infarction. These causes produce either temporary or permanent heart block.

Significance: CHF may develop in infancy, particularly when there is associated CHD. Patients with isolated congenital heart block are usually asymptomatic during childhood. Syncopal attacks

(Stokes-Adams attack) or sudden death may occur with the heart rate below 40 to 45 beats/min.

Treatment

a. No treatment is required for asymptomatic children with congenital complete heart block. Atropine or isoproterenol is used in symptomatic children and adults until temporary ventricular pacing is secured.

b. A temporary transvenous ventricular pacemaker is indicated for patients with possible transient heart block or prophylactically for patients who might develop heart block. Permanent artificial ventricular pacemaker is indicated for patients with surgically induced heart block and those with congenital heart block who are symptomatic or who have CHF (see Chapter 6 for the newborn with complete heart block).

NEWBORNS WITH CARDIAC PROBLEMS

VI

In the cardiac evaluation of the newborn, understanding the circulatory status at birth is very important. As the result of fetal circulation, newborn infants have RV dominance with a thick RV wall and elevated pulmonary vascular resistance (PVR) with a thick medial layer of the pulmonary arterioles. The thick pulmonary artery smooth muscle gradually becomes thinner, and it resembles that of the adult by the time the baby is age 6 to 8 weeks. Most perinatal changes in hemodynamics are related to the thinning of the pulmonary vascular smooth muscle, resulting in a gradual fall in the PVR and a loss of RV dominance of the newborn. Premature infants in general have less RV dominance than full-term infants, and the PVR is not as high as in the full-term neonate, which adds variability to the process. Because of these unique aspects of the perinatal circulatory system, the basic tools in the initial cardiac evaluation discussed in Chapter 1 are less reliable and the findings may be different in the newborn. Therefore echo studies are commonly performed in the neonatal cardiac evaluation. Some important aspects of normal and abnormal findings in physical examination, ECG, and CXR films of the newborn are briefly reviewed in this chapter.

I. INITIAL EVALUATION OF THE NEWBORN

A. Physical Examination

1. Normal physical findings that are unique in normal newborn infants

   a. Heart rate is generally faster (usually over 100 beats/min, with normal ranges from 70 to 180 beats/min) than that of older children and adults.

   b. A varying degree of acrocyanosis is the rule rather than the exception.

   c. Mild arterial desaturation with arterial Po_2 as low as 60 mm Hg is not unusual in an otherwise normal neonate. This may be caused by an intrapulmonary shunt through an as yet unexpanded portion of the lungs or by a right-to-left atrial shunt through the patent foramen ovale (PFO).

   d. There is relative hyperactivity of the RV, with the point of maximal impulse (PMI) at the LLSB rather than at the apex.

   e. The S2 may be single in the first days of life, and occasionally an ejection click (reflecting pulmonary hypertension) is audible.

   f. An innocent heart murmur may be present. The most common one in this age group is the pulmonary flow murmur of the newborn.

   g. Peripheral pulses are easily palpable in all extremities, including the foot, in *every* normal infant.

2. Additional important features of premature infants

   a. The pulmonary flow murmur of the newborn is more frequent and louder in premature than in full-term infants.

   b. The likelihood of a PDA murmur is greater in premature infants.

   c. The peripheral pulses normally appear bounding because of the lack of a normal amount of subcutaneous tissue.

3. Abnormal physical findings

The following abnormal physical findings suggest cardiac pathology.

   a. Cyanosis, particularly when it does not improve with oxygen administration, requires further evaluation.

   b. Decreased or absent peripheral pulses in the lower extremities suggest COA. Generally weak peripheral pulses suggest hypoplastic left heart syndrome (HLHS) or circulatory shock. Bounding peripheral pulses suggest an aortic runoff lesion such as PDA or persistent truncus arteriosus.

c. Tachypnea of greater than 60 breaths/min with or without retraction is abnormal.

d. Hepatomegaly may suggest a heart defect manifesting with CHF. A midline liver suggests asplenia or polysplenia syndrome.

e. A heart murmur may be a presenting sign of CHD. However, innocent murmurs are more common than pathologic murmurs.

f. An irregular rhythm or abnormal heart rate may suggest cardiac arrhythmias.

g. Blood pressure readings in the lower extremities 6 to 7 mm Hg lower than those in the arm require further evaluation for COA.

B. Electrocardiography

1. The normal ECG of a newborn is different from that of a child or an adult as follows:

   a. Sinus tachycardia with a rate as high as 180 beats/min.

   b. A rightward QRS axis with a mean of +125 degrees and a maximum of +180 degrees.

   c. Relatively small voltages for the QRS complex and the T wave.

   d. RV dominance with tall R waves in the RPLs (V4R, V1, and V2).

   e. Occasional q waves in V1 (seen in about 10% of normal newborns).

   f. Benign arrhythmias.

2. An abnormal ECG may be in the form of an abnormal P axis, abnormal QRS axis, hypertrophy of the ventricles or atria, ventricular conduction disturbances, or arrhythmias. Because of the wide ranges of normal values, many newborn infants with significant CHDs may show a normal ECG for their age. Arrhythmias in the newborn are discussed later in this chapter.

a. P axis
   1) A P axis in the right lower quadrant (+90 to +180 degrees) suggests atrial situs inversus, asplenia syndrome, or incorrectly placed ECG electrodes.
   2) A superior P axis suggests an ectopic atrial rhythm, as seen in polysplenia syndrome.
b. QRS axis
   1) A superiorly oriented QRS axis between 0 and −150 degrees (left anterior hemiblock) suggests partial or complete ECD, including splenic syndromes, or tricuspid atresia.
   2) A QRS axis less than +30 degrees is abnormal and indicates left axis deviation (LAD) in the newborn. The QRS axis between +30 and +60 degrees is unusual and indicates relative LAD.
   3) A QRS axis greater than +180 degrees (in the range of −150 to −180 degrees) may indicate RAD.
c. LVH is suggested in the newborn when the following are present:
   1) LAD or relative LAD (less than +60 degrees) for the newborn.
   2) An R/S progression in the precordial leads that resembles the adult R/S progression.
   3) QRS voltages demonstrating abnormal leftward and posterior forces or abnormal inferior forces for age (see Chapter 1 for normal values).
d. RVH is difficult to diagnose because of the normal dominance of the RV at this age. However, the following are helpful clues to RVH in the newborn.
   1) S waves in lead I 12 mm or greater.
   2) Pure R waves with no S waves in V1 greater than 10 mm.
   3) R waves in V1 greater than 25 mm or R waves in aVR greater than 8 mm.
   4) A qR pattern in V1 (this is also seen in 10% of normal newborns).
   5) Upright T waves in V1 after 3 days of age.

      6) RAD with the QRS axis greater than +180 degrees.

  e. Atrial hypertrophy

    1) Right atrial hypertrophy (RAH) is present when P wave amplitude is greater than 3 mm in any lead.

    2) Left atrial hypertrophy (LAH) is present when P wave duration is 0.08 sec or greater (usually with notched P waves in the limb leads and biphasic P waves in V1).

  f. Ventricular conduction disturbances (i.e., RBBB, LBBB, WPW syndrome, and intraventricular block) are present when the QRS duration is 0.07 sec or more (not 0.1 sec or greater as in the adult) (see Fig 1-21).

    1) RBBB may be associated with Ebstein anomaly and COA in the newborn. It is sometimes seen in otherwise normal neonates.

    2) LBBB is extremely rare in the newborn.

    3) Intraventricular block (with a widening of the QRS complex throughout the QRS duration) is more significant than RBBB because it is often associated with significant metabolic abnormalities (e.g., hypoxia, acidosis, hyperkalemia) and diffuse myocardial diseases.

    4) WPW syndrome may be an isolated finding or may be associated with CHDs such as Ebstein anomaly or L-TGA. It is a frequent cause of SVT.

C. Chest Roentgenography

  1. Normal CXR findings

    a. The cardiothoracic (CT) ratio of normal newborn infants may be greater than 0.5 because of inadequate inspiration and a large thymic shadow.

    b. The thymic shadow may have any of several shapes, including a classic sail sign, or may have undulant or smooth borders, either unilateral or bilateral, on the upper mediastinum.

    c. Cardiac silhouette is not always as well defined in neonates as in older children.

    d. Evaluation of pulmonary vascular markings in the neonate poses a special problem. Although a reduced PBF is usually easier to detect (and indicates serious cyanotic CHD), increased vascularity is not always apparent even when the pulmonary blood flow is large. The distinction between increased PBF and pulmonary venous congestion is often difficult.

2. Abnormal CXR findings: A cardiac problem is suggested by an abnormal size, position, or silhouette of the heart, by an abnormal shape or position of the liver, and by increased or decreased pulmonary vascularity on CXR films.

    a. Heart size

      The CT ratio is of limited value, since that of normal neonates is usually greater than 0.5. Many serious CHDs that eventually result in cardiomegaly show a normal heart size in the newborn. Unequivocal cardiomegaly may be due to CHD (such as VSD, PDA, TGA, Ebstein anomaly, HLHS, and others), myocarditis or cardiomyopathy, pericardial effusion, metabolic disturbances (e.g., hypoglycemia, severe hypoxemia, and acidosis), and overhydration or overtransfusion.

      In the newborn who is intubated and on a ventilator, the heart size is greatly influenced by the ventilator setting. For example, a premature infant with a large-shunt PDA may have a normal-sized heart on CXR film if the ventilator settings are high, especially the positive end-expiratory pressure.

    b. Abnormal cardiac silhouettes may be of considerable help in suggesting the correct diagnosis (see Fig 1-30).

      1) A boot-shaped heart (*coeur en sabot*) is seen in TOF and in tricuspid atresia.

      2) An egg-shaped heart with narrow waist may be seen in TGA.

      3) A large, globular heart is seen in Ebstein anomaly.

    c. Dextrocardia or mesocardia

      The presence of dextrocardia or mesocardia does

not always indicate a serious heart defect. The segmental approach should be used for further evaluation. Four common situations seen in dextrocardia or situs inversus totalis are situs inversus totalis with a normal heart, a rightward displacement of normally formed heart due to hypoplasia of the right lung, a complex cyanotic CHD, and asplenia or polysplenia syndrome.

d. The situs of abdominal viscera: A left-sided liver with the heart in the right side of the chest is seen in situs inversus totalis with normal heart. The liver and the cardiac apex on the same side suggest a complex cyanotic CHD. A midline liver suggests asplenia or polysplenia syndrome.

e. Pulmonary vascular markings

1) Increased PVMs in a cyanotic infant suggest TGA, persistent truncus arteriosus, or single ventricle. In an acyanotic infant, increased PVMs suggest VSD, PDA, or ECD.

2) Decreased PVMs suggest a critical cyanotic CHD with decreased PBF, such as pulmonary atresia, tricuspid atresia, or TOF with severe pulmonary stenosis or atresia.

3) A ground-glass appearance or a reticulated pattern of the lung fields is characteristic of pulmonary venous obstruction (seen with HLHS or TAPVR with obstruction).

II. PROBLEM-BASED APPROACHES

The majority of cardiology consultations for newborns are requested for one or more of the following reasons: heart murmur, cyanosis, abnormal CXR findings, abnormal ECGs, possible CHF, and cardiac arrhythmias. Abnormal ECG or CXR findings are discussed earlier in this chapter.

A. Heart Murmurs

1. Innocent heart murmurs: More than 50% of full-term newborn infants (and a higher percentage of premature infants) have an innocent systolic murmur at

some time during the first week of life. Infants with innocent heart murmurs have normal ECG and CXR findings. The four most common innocent murmurs in the newborn period are as follows:

a. Pulmonary flow murmur is most common. It is more often found in premature and small-for-gestational-age infants than in full-term infants. A soft systolic murmur (grade 1 to 2/6), heard best at the ULSB, transmits well to both sides of the chest, axillae, and the back.

b. Transient systolic murmur of PDA is soft (grade 1 to 2/6) is audible at the ULSB and in the left infraclavicular area on the first day. It usually disappears shortly thereafter.

c. Transient systolic murmur of tricuspid regurgitation is indistinguishable from that of VSD and is most common in infants who had fetal distress or neonatal asphyxia.

d. Vibratory systolic innocent murmur is a counterpart of Still murmur in older children.

2. Pathologic heart murmurs: Most pathologic murmurs except ASD are audible during the first month of life. The time of appearance of a murmur depends on the nature of the defect.

a. Heart murmurs of stenotic lesions (e.g., AS, PS) are audible immediately after birth and persist.

b. Heart murmurs of L-R shunt lesions, especially those of a large VSD, may appear later, when the PVR decreases. The murmur of ASD appears late in infancy or in childhood.

c. The continuous murmur of a large PDA may not appear for 2 to 3 weeks. Instead, it is a crescendo systolic murmur with a slight or no diastolic component.

Even in the absence of a murmur, a newborn infant may have a serious heart defect that requires immediate attention, e.g., severe cyanotic heart disease such as TGA or pulmonary atresia with a closing PDA. Infants who are in severe CHF may not have a loud murmur until the myocardial function is improved with anticongestive measures.

B. Cyanosis in the Newborn

Most patients with severe forms of CHD have cyanosis at birth. Early detection of cyanosis in a newborn is crucial. When in doubt, blood gases for Po_2 or transcutaneous oxygen saturation should be obtained to confirm or rule out central cyanosis. Normal 1-day-old infants may have a Po_2 as low as 60 mm Hg, but oxygen saturation is higher than 90% because of the normally leftward oxygen hemoglobin dissociation curve.

1. Central cyanosis (with arterial desaturation or decreased arterial Po_2) may be due to central nervous system depression, lung disease, or cyanotic CHD. Table 6-1 lists some of the causes and characteristic physical and laboratory findings of each type of cyanosis. Cyanosis associated with normal arterial oxygen saturation (or normal Po_2) is called peripheral cyanosis and is less important than central cyanosis. Examples of peripheral cyanosis include acrocyanosis, exposure to cold, and decreased peripheral perfusion.

2. Suggested approach to neonates with central cyanosis
   a. CXR films may reveal pulmonary causes of cyanosis and urgency of the problem. They will also hint at the presence and the type of any cardiac defects.
   b. Arterial blood gases on room air will confirm or rule out central cyanosis. Elevated Pco_2 suggests pulmonary or CNS problems. Low pH may be seen in sepsis, circulatory shock, or severe hypoxemia.
   c. Hyperoxitest: repeating arterial blood gases while breathing 100% oxygen helps to separate cardiac causes of cyanosis from pulmonary or CNS causes. With pulmonary or CNS diseases, arterial Po_2 usually rises to more than 100 mm Hg. When there is a significant intracardiac R-L shunt, the arterial Po_2 does not exceed 100 mm Hg, and the rise is usually not more than 10 to 30 mm Hg with cyanotic CHD.
   d. Obtain an ECG if cardiac origin of cyanosis is suspected.
   e. Umbilical artery line: A Po_2 value in a preductal artery (such as right radial artery) higher than that

TABLE 6-1.

Causes and Clinical Characteristics of Central Cyanosis

A. CNS depression

Causes: Perinatal asphyxia, heavy maternal sedation, intrauterine fetal distress, etc.

Findings: Shallow irregular respiration, poor muscle tone. Cyanosis disappears when the infant is stimulated or given oxygen.

B. Pulmonary disease

Causes: Parenchymal lung disease (e.g., hyaline membrane disease, atelectasis), pneumothorax or pleural effusion, diaphragmatic hernia, and PPHN (or PFC syndrome).

Findings: Tachypnea and respiratory distress with retraction and expiratory grunting, rales, or decreased breath sounds on auscultation; CXRs may reveal causes (as listed above). Oxygen administration improves or abolishes cyanosis.

C. Cardiac disease

Causes: Cyanotic CHD with R–L shunt.

Findings: Tachypnea, usually without retraction. No rales or abnormal breath sounds unless CHF supervenes.

Heart murmur may be absent in serious forms of cyanotic CHD.

A continuous murmur (of PDA) may indicate restricted PBF through the ductus.

CXRs may show cardiomegaly, abnormal cardiac silhouette, increased or decreased PVM.

Little or no increase in Po_2 with oxygen administration.

PPHN, persistent pulmonary hypertension of the newborn; PFC, persistence of fetal circulation.

in a postductal artery (umbilical artery line) by 10 to 15 mm Hg suggests an R-L shunt through a PDA. Such a differential Po_2 level may result from persistent pulmonary hypertension of the newborn (PPHN), critical AS, interrupted aortic arch, or coarctation of the aorta. An echo study will clarify the cause of the differential Po_2 levels.

f. Prostaglandin E_1: If a cyanotic CHD is suspected after these laboratory tests, PGE_1 (alprostadil, Prostin VR Pediatric) should be started or made available. The starting dose is 0.05 to 0.1 µg/kg/

min, administered in a continuous IV drip. When the desired effects (increased Po_2, increased systemic blood pressure, and improved pH) are achieved, the dose should be reduced step-by-step to 0.01 µg/kg/min. When there is no effect with the initial starting dose, it may be increased to 0.4 µg/kg/min. Three common side effects of PGE_1 IV infusion are apnea (12%), fever (14%), and flushing (10%).

g. Cardiology consultation is called for if cardiac origin of cyanosis is suspected.

Discussion of individual cyanotic heart defects is in Chapter 3. Only PPHN will be discussed in this section.

Persistent Pulmonary Hypertension of the Newborn (Persistence of the Fetal Circulation, or PFC Syndrome)

Prevalence: PPHN occurs in approximately 1 in 1500 live births.

Pathology and Pathophysiology: This condition of neonates is characterized by the persistence of pulmonary hypertension, which in turn causes a varying degree of cyanosis from an R-L shunt through the PDA or the PFO. No underlying CHD is present. Various causes have been identified, and they can be divided into three groups by the anatomy of the pulmonary vascular bed.

1. *Intense pulmonary vasoconstriction in the presence of normally developed pulmonary vascular bed.* Clinical conditions such as perinatal asphyxia, meconium aspiration, ventricular dysfunction, group B streptococcal pneumonia, hyperviscosity syndrome, and hypoglycemia are frequent causes of pulmonary vasoconstriction. Alveolar hypoxia and acidosis are also important causes of pulmonary vasoconstriction. Thromboxane, vasoconstrictor prostaglandins, leukotrienes, and endothelin may also play an important role in pulmonary vasoconstriction.

2. *Hypertrophy (of the medial layer) of the pulmonary arterioles.* Chronic intrauterine hypoxia and maternal ingestion of nonsteroidal antiinflammatory agents are

important causes of pulmonary arteriolar hypertrophy.

3. *Developmentally abnormal pulmonary arterioles with decreased cross-sectional area of the pulmonary vascular bed.* Congenital diaphragmatic hernia and primary pulmonary hypoplasia are examples.

In general, pulmonary hypertension secondary to the first group is easier to reverse than that caused by the second group. Pulmonary hypertension caused by the third group is most difficult or even impossible to reverse.

Varying degrees of myocardial dysfunction often accompany PPHN. These abnormalities are caused by global and/or subendocardial ischemia (and aggravated by hypoglycemia and hypocalcemia).

Clinical Manifestations

1. Full-term or postterm neonates are most often affected. History of meconium staining, birth asphyxia, or maternal ingestion of nonsteroidal antiinflammatory agents (in the third trimester) may be present.

2. Cyanosis and tachypnea with grunting and retraction develop 6 to 12 hours after birth. The S2 is loud and single, with a prominent RV impulse. A soft systolic murmur of TR, systemic hypotension, or even CHF may be present.

3. The arterial Po_2 is lower in the descending aorta or legs than in the right arm (because of an R-L ductal shunt) and differential cyanosis may be evident (with pink upper body and cyanotic lower part of the body). No difference in Po_2 at the two sites may be the result of an R-L shunt predominantly at the atrial level.

4. The ECG is usually normal for age, but occasional RVH or T wave changes suggestive of myocardial dysfunction may be present.

5. CXR film reveals varying degrees of cardiomegaly with or without findings suggestive of meconium aspiration.

6. Echo studies show no evidence of cyanotic CHD but

do show a large PDA. An R-L shunt is detected by the Doppler study at the ductal level or atrial level (PFO or ASD). CHD such as COA or interrupted aortic arch should be ruled out.

Treatment: Three goals of therapy are (1) to lower the PVR by administration of oxygen and pulmonary vasodilators (such as tolazoline) and sometimes induction of respiratory alkalosis by the use of a ventilator, (2) to correct myocardial dysfunction (by dopamine, dobutamine), and (3) to stabilize the patient and treat associated conditions (e.g., acidosis, hypocalcemia, hypoglycemia).

Inhaled nitric oxide (NO) is promising in lowering the pulmonary artery pressure. Extracorporeal membrane oxygenation (ECMO) is effective in selected patients with severe PPHN.

C. Heart Failure in the Newborn

The clinical picture of CHF in the newborn may simulate another disorder such as meningitis, sepsis, pneumonia, or bronchiolitis. Tachypnea, tachycardia, pulmonary rales or rhonchi, hepatomegaly, and weak peripheral pulses are common presenting signs. Heart murmur is either faint or absent. Cardiomegaly on CXR film is always present, with or without increased PVMs or pulmonary edema. Causes of CHF in the newborn are listed in Table 6-2. The time of onset of CHF varies rather predictably with the type of CHD. Detailed discussion of treatment of CHF is presented in Chapter 7.

Two important CHDs that present with CHF in the newborn period are hypoplastic left heart syndrome (HLHS) and large PDA in premature infants. Transient myocardial ischemia and diabetes in the mother are other causes of CHF in the newborn. These four conditions are presented in this chapter.

Hypoplastic Left Heart Syndrome

Prevalence: HLHS occurs in 1% of all CHDs and is the most common cause of death from CHD during the first month of life.

TABLE 6-2.

Causes of Heart Failure in the Newborn

A. Structural heart defects
    At birth
        Hypoplastic left heart syndrome (HLHS)
        Severe tricuspid or pulmonary regurgitation
        Large systemic AV fistula
    Week 1
        TGA
        Large PDA in premature infant
        TAPVR below diaphragm
    Weeks 1–4
        Critical AS or PS
        Preductal COA
B. Noncardiac causes
    1. Birth asphyxia (resulting in transient myocardial ischemia)
    2. Metabolic: hypoglycemia, hypocalcemia
    3. Severe anemia (as seen in hydrops fetalis)
    4. Neonatal sepsis
    5. Overtransfusion or overhydration
C. Primary myocardial disease
    1. Myocarditis
    2. Transient myocardial ischemia (with or without birth
       asphyxia)
    3. Cardiomyopathy (seen in infants of diabetic mothers)
D. Disturbances in heart rate
    1. Supraventricular tachycardia (SVT or PAT)
    2. Atrial flutter or fibrillation
    3. Congenital heart block (when associated with CHD)

Pathology and Pathophysiology

1. HLHS includes a group of closely related anomalies characterized by hypoplasia of the LV (from atresia or severe stenosis of the aortic and/or mitral valves) and hypoplasia of the ascending aorta and aortic arch. The LA is small, and the atrial septum is frequently intact other than the PFO.

2. During fetal life the PVR is higher than the SVR, and the dominant RV maintains normal perfusing pressure in the descending aorta through the ductal R-L shunt, even in the presence of the nonfunctioning hy-

poplastic LV. However, difficulties arise after birth, primarily from two factors: (1) reversal of the vascular resistance in the two circuits with the SVR higher than the PVR, and (2) closure of the PDA. The end result is a marked decrease in systemic cardiac output and aortic pressure, resulting in circulatory shock and metabolic acidosis. An increase in PBF in the presence of the nonfunctioning LV results in an elevated LA pressure and pulmonary edema.

Clinical Manifestations

1. The neonate is critically ill in the first few hours to days of life, with mild cyanosis, tachycardia, tachypnea, and pulmonary rales.
2. Poor peripheral pulses and vasoconstricted extremities are characteristic. The S2 is loud and single. Heart murmur is usually absent, but a grade 1 to 3/6 ejection systolic murmur may be present over the precordium.
3. The ECG shows RVH. Rarely, LVH is present because V5 and V6 leads are obtained over the dilated RV.
4. CXR films show pulmonary venous congestion or pulmonary edema. The heart is only mildly enlarged.
5. The arterial blood gas determination reveals severe metabolic acidosis in the presence of a slightly decreased Po_2, a characteristic finding of this condition.
6. Echo findings are diagnostic and usually obviate cardiac catheterization. Severe hypoplasia of the aorta and aortic annulus and the absent or distorted mitral valve are usually imaged. The LV cavity is diminutive. The RV cavity is markedly dilated, and the tricuspid valve is large. A partially constricted PDA may be imaged.
7. Progressive hypoxemia and acidosis result in death usually in the first month of life.

Management

Medical

a. Intubation, administration of oxygen, and correction of metabolic acidosis are important.
b. An IV infusion of PGE_1 may produce temporary improvement by reopening the ductus arteriosus.

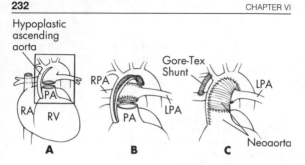

Hypoplastic
ascending
aorta

FIG. 6-1.
Schematic diagram of Norwood procedure. **A,** The heart with aortic
atresia and a hypoplastic ascending aorta and aortic arch are shown.
The MPA is transected. **B,** The distal PA is closed with a patch. An
incision is made in the ascending aorta that extends around the
aortic arch to the level of the ductus. The ductus is ligated. **C,** A
modified right Blalock-Taussig shunt is created between the right
subclavian artery and the RPA as the sole source of pulmonary blood
flow. Using an aortic (or pulmonary arterial) allograft (shaded area),
the PA is anastomosed to the ascending aorta and the aortic arch
to create a large arterial trunk. The procedure to widen the atrial
communication is not shown.

      c. Balloon atrial septostomy during a cardiac cath-
         eterization may help decompress the LA and im-
         prove oxygenation but will be only a temporary
         benefit.
       Surgical: Three options are available in the manage-
         ment of these infants: do nothing or choose one of
         two surgical options. The surgical options are the
         Norwood operation (followed by a Fontan opera-
         tion) and cardiac transplantation. Surgical proce-
         dure of choice remains controversial.
  1. Norwood operation
    a. The first-stage Norwood operation (Fig 6-1) is per-
       formed on the neonate. This operation consists of
       (1) division of the MPA and closure of the distal
       stump, (2) a right-sided Gore-Tex shunt (usually 4

mm tube) to provide PBF, (3) the excision of the atrial septum (for adequate interatrial mixing), and (4) construction of a new aortic arch between the proximal MPA and the hypoplastic ascending aorta and aortic arch, using an aortic or pulmonary artery allograft. The surgical mortality rate is 35% or higher.

b. A cavopulmonary shunt (or bidirectional Glenn operation) (see Fig 3-13, *A*) is carried out at 6 months of age. Mortality is less than 5%.

c. A modified Fontan operation is carried out when the patient is a year and a half old (see Fig 3-13, *B*). Overall survival after the Fontan operation is about 50% at 4 years.

2. Cardiac transplantation is considered to be the procedure of choice in some centers. The transplantation is not a cure for the defect but creates a lifelong medical problem, the threat of infection and rejection.

Premature Newborns with Large PDA

Prevalence: Significant PDA with CHF occurs in 15% of prematures with birth weight less than 1,750 g and in 40% to 50% of those with birth weight less than 1,500 g.

Pathophysiology: This is a special problem in premature infants who have been recovering from hyaline membrane disease. With improvement in oxygenation the PVR drops rapidly, but the ductus remains patent because its responsiveness to oxygen is immature in the premature newborn. The resulting large L-R ductal shunt makes the lungs stiff, and weaning the infant from ventilator and oxygen therapy becomes difficult. Infants who remain on ventilators for a long time develop bronchopulmonary dysplasia with resulting pulmonary hypertension (cor pulmonale) and right heart failure.

Clinical Manifestations

1. History usually reveals that a premature infant with hyaline membrane disease has made some improvement during the first few days after birth, but this is followed by inability to wean the infant from the

ventilator or a need to increase ventilator settings or oxygen requirement in 4- to 7-day-old premature infants. Apneic spells or episodes of bradycardia may be initial signs in infants who are not on ventilators.

2. Bounding peripheral pulses and hyperactive precordium are usually present. The classic continuous murmur of PDA at the ULSB is diagnostic, but the murmur is sometimes only systolic at the middle and upper LSB. Premature infants who are fluid-overloaded or retaining fluid may also present with the hyperdynamic precordium, an ejection systolic murmur, a bounding pulse, and a wide pulse pressure.

3. The ECG is usually normal.

4. CXR films show cardiomegaly and evidence of pulmonary edema or pulmonary venous congestion in addition to varying degrees of the lung disease.

5. 2D echo study confirms the diagnosis. It provides the anatomic information about the diameter, length, and shape of the ductus. The Doppler study of the ductus (with the sample volume placed at the pulmonary end of the ductus) provides important functional information such as ductal shunt patterns (pure L-R, bidirectional, or predominant R-L shunt), pressures in the PA, and magnitude of the ductal shunt or pulmonary perfusion status. An indirect estimate of the magnitude of the shunt can be made by the LA and LV dimensions.

Management: For symptomatic infants, either pharmacologic (indomethacin) or surgical closure of the ductus is indicated. A small PDA that is not causing CHF should be followed up medically for 6 months without surgical ligation because of the possibility of spontaneous closure.

1. Indomethacin (a prostaglandin synthetase inhibitor) 0.2 mg/kg IV every 12 hours up to three doses may be used on selected cases. Contraindications to the use of indomethacin include (1) BUN over 25 mg/dl or creatinine levels over 1.8 mg/dl, (2) a platelet count below 80,000/mm^3, (3) a bleeding tendency (including intracranial hemorrhage), (4) necrotizing enterocolitis, and (5) hyperbilirubinemia.

2. If indomethacin is unsuccessful or if the use of indomethacin is contraindicated, surgical ligation of the ductus is indicated.

Transient Myocardial Ischemia

Prevalence: Transient myocardial ischemia is a rarely recognized condition; the prevalence is unknown.

Pathology and Pathophysiology

1. Subendocardial ischemia or necrosis (possibly secondary to hypoxic pulmonary vasoconstriction) occurs in the papillary muscles and other areas of the ventricles in the newborn who had prenatal or perinatal hypoxia and distress. Evidence of pulmonary hypertension, bidirectional shunts at the atrial and/or ductal levels, and TR are usually present. Variable degrees of LV dysfunction are demonstrable by echo.

2. Three levels of severity have been recognized.
   a. *Transient tachypnea of the newborn* is the mildest form of the condition. Mild LV dysfunction leads to fluid retention, pulmonary edema and reduced lung compliance producing tachypnea.
   b. Transient tricuspid (or mitral) regurgitation results from papillary muscle infarction (evidenced by elevated serum levels of creatine phosphokinase [CPK] MB fraction).
   c. Severe CHF with cardiogenic shock is the most severe form of myocardial dysfunction seen in the newborn.

Clinical Manifestations

1. Tachypnea develops usually in full-term neonates with a low Apgar score. Mild cyanosis may also be present.

2. A systolic murmur of TR or MR is commonly present. Rarely, CHF with gallop rhythm, hypotension, and vascular collapse result.

3. The ECG may show generalized flat T waves and minor ST segment depression. Abnormal Q waves suggestive of anterior or inferior infarction may be seen.

4. CXR films show varying degrees, sometimes marked, of cardiomegaly. PVMs may be increased due to pulmonary venous congestion (described as wet lung) in severly affected neonates.

5. Echo reveals varying degrees of myocardial dysfunction, including an enlarged LA and/or LV, decreased contractility of the LV, and MR.

6. Laboratory studies may reveal mild reduction of P_{O_2} and pH (but usually without CO_2 retention), hypoglycemia, and elevated CPK MB fraction in patients with significant TR. A myocardial perfusion scan may show a diffuse impairment of thallium-201 uptake (different from myocarditis, in which myocardial perfusion is normal).

7. Infants with transient myocardial ischemia usually recover unless it is associated with severe acidosis, CNS damages, or advanced sepsis.

Management

1. Supportive measures with administration of oxygen, correction of acidosis, and treatment of hypoglycemia are all that are required for mild cases.

2. For severely affected infants, ventilatory assistance, short-acting inotropic agents (such as dopamine), a vasodilator agent, and fluid restriction and diuretic(s) may be indicated.

Infants of Diabetic Mothers

Prevalence: At least 1.3% of pregnancies are complicated by diabetes mellitus.

Pathology

1. Congenital malformations of all types are increased (three to four times those found in the general population). Neural tube defects (anencephaly, myelomeningocele), CHDs, and sacral dysgenesis or agenesis are common.

2. There is a high prevalence of CHDs, cardiomyopathy, and PPHN in these infants.
   a. The risk of CHD is also three to four times as great as in the general population, with VSD, TGA, and COA among the more common defects.
   b. Hypertrophic cardiomyopathy with or without obstruction is seen in 10% to 20% of these infants. Cardiac hypertrophy is considered to be caused by hyperinsulinemia.

    c. There is an increased risk of PPHN, which may be in part related to conditions that promote the persistence of pulmonary hypertension such as hypoglycemia, perinatal asphyxia, respiratory distress, and polycythemia.

Clinical Manifestations: Clinical manifestations of only the cardiomyopathy will be presented.

1. History usually reveals gestational or insulin-dependent diabetes mellitus in the mother. Progressive respiratory distress with tachypnea from birth is often present.

2. These large-for-gestational-age babies are often plethoric and mildly cyanotic, and they may have tachypnea (80 to 100 breaths/min) and tachycardia (above 160 beats/min). Signs of CHF with gallop rhythm may be present in 5% to 10% of these babies. There may be a systolic murmur along the LSB, which may be due to LVOT obstruction or associated CHD.

3. CXR film may reveal varying degrees of cardiomegaly. PVMs are either normal or mildly increased because of pulmonary venous congestion.

4. The ECG is usually nonspecific, but a long QT interval (a long ST segment due to hypocalcemia) may be present. Occasionally, RVH, LVH, or CVH is seen.

5. Echo may show asymmetric septal hypertrophy (ASH, with disproportionately thicker septum than the LV posterior wall), but even the posterior walls are also thicker than normal. Supernormal contractility of the LV and evidence of LVOT obstruction (systolic anterior motion [SAM] of the mitral valve and fluttering of the aortic valve) are present in about 50% of these infants. Rarely, the LV is dilated and its contractility decreased.

6. In most cases the hypertrophy spontaneously resolves within the first 6 to 12 months of life.

Treatment

1. General supportive measures such as IV fluids, correction of hypoglycemia and hypocalcemia, and ventilatory assistance, if indicated.

2. β-Adrenergic blockers such as propranolol may be helpful for the LVOT obstruction, but the treatment is usually not necessary. Digitalis and other inotropic agents are contraindicated, since they may worsen the obstruction.

3. If the LV is dilated with decreased LV contractility, usual anticongestive measures (with digoxin, diuretics) are indicated.

D. Arrhythmias and AV Conduction Disturbances of the Newborn

Holter Monitoring in the Newborn

Monitoring of the cardiac rhythm in an intensive care setting has allowed us to detect many types of arrhythmias and condution disturbances that are not ordinarily recorded on the routine ECG and rhythm strips. Frequent use of long-term recording (Holter monitoring) of cardiac rhythm has resulted in better understanding of the frequency and nature of arrhythmias throughout the day. Arrhythmias of the newborn must be interpreted within the context of the findings of the long-term ECG monitoring. Results from several recent studies on healthy newborns are summarized below.

1. In full-term newborns the highest heart rate was 230 beats/min and the lowest sinus rate was as low as 75 beats/min. Premature atrial contraction (PAC) (10% to 35%), junctional rhythm (25%), and sinus pause (up to 72%) were common in normal newborns. PVCs (1% to 13%), SVTs (4%), and 2:1 sinus node exit block were occasionally present.

2. In preterm and low-birth-weight newborns, the fastest and slowest heart rates were 210 and 75 beats/min, respectively. PACs (2% to 33%), PVCs (6% to 17%), junctional rhythm (18% to 70%), and sudden sinus bradycardia below 90 beats/min (up to 90%) were common. Sudden sinus arrest of up to 2 seconds was seen in 6% and sinus arrhythmias in 100% of preterm newborns. Bradyarrhythmias are seen more commonly in preterm than in term infants.

Basic Arrhythmias

This section discusses significance and management of only well-defined arrhythmias seen in the newborn. Detailed discussion of arrhythmias and AV conduction disturbances is in Chapter 5.

The definitions of tachycardia and bradycardia for the adult and older child do not apply to the newborn. Normal resting heart rate of the newborn is 110 to 150 beats/min, but depending on the state of sleep or activity, the rate ranges from 80 to 190 beats/min. Rates persistently above or below this range require investigation.

Sinus Tachycardia: Transient tachycardia up to 180 to 190 beats/min is commonly seen in normal newborns and does not require treatment, but the maximal rate usually does not exceed 220 beats/min. Persistent tachycardia may be caused by hypovolemia, hyperthermia, administration of catecholamines or theophylline, or hyperthyroidism. Treatment should be directed toward detection and correction of the underlying cause.

Sinus Bradycardia: A heart rate persistently below 80 beats/min in a newborn infant may be called bradycardia. Transient bradycardia (below 70 beats/min) may be seen in normal neonates and requires no treatment. Prolonged bradycardia may either precede or follow apnea, maternal medications (such as reserpine), or neonatal asphyxia. Treatment should be directed to correct or improve underlying causes.

Sinus Arrhythmia: Sinus arrhythmia is quite common in healthy full-term and premature infants. Unlike a similar variation in older children, it may or may not be related to respiration. It has no clinical significance.

Sinus Pause or Arrest: Occasionally a normal full-term or premature neonate has sinus pause or arrest, but digitalis toxicity or hyperkalemia should be considered as possibilities.

Premature Atrial Contraction: PAC is common in healthy newborns. It is also seen in infants with heart defects, after cardiac surgery, and in digitalis toxicity. Many nonconducted PACs may result in a low heart rate. Usually no treatment is indicated except for infants with digitalis toxicity.

Supraventricular Tachycardia: There are three mechanisms for SVT. Reciprocating AV tachycardia is the most frequent. Nonreciprocating atrial tachycardia and nodal tachycardia are rare forms (see Chapter 5).

SVT is characterized by rapid heart rates, usually 200 to 300 beats/min, with the QRS complex of normal duration. The episodes usually start and end abruptly. WPW syndrome is responsible in about 50% of SVTs in the neonate. Structural heart diseases (such as Ebstein anomaly, tricuspid atresia, and cardiac tumors) are less frequent causes. Viral myocarditis and thyrotoxicosis have been associated with SVT as well. Short episodes of tachycardia are well tolerated. Newborns with sustained SVT become restless and tachypneic and have feeding difficulties, eventually developing signs of CHF and circulatory shock.

Adenosine is the treatment of choice, followed by digitals. It is given in a rapid IV bolus, starting at 50 µg/kg and increasing in increments of 50 µg/kg, every 1 to 2 min (maximum 250 µg/kg). If the baby is unresponsive to adenosine and CHF is present, cardioversion may be performed followed by digitalization and diuretics. In SVT of short duration without signs of CHF, digoxin alone is used. Application of an ice bag to the face has been employed successfully in some neonates. Vagal stimulatory maneuvers are rarely effective in neonates. Transesophageal atrial overdrive stimulation may be effective. Neither verapamil nor propranolol is the drug of choice; one or the other is tried only when other measures fail. These drugs may produce extreme bradycardia and hypotension in the newborn.

Atrial Flutter or Fibrillation: A relatively rare arrhythmia, atrial flutter or fibrillation is often associated with CHD (such as Ebstein anomaly, MS, tricuspid atresia), viral myocarditis, and systemic infections. Severe CHF may develop if the ventricular response is very fast. Cardioversion followed by digoxin is the treatment of choice for infants who are in CHF. In the infant without CHF, the use of digoxin is indicated to prevent CHF by keeping the ventricular rate within an acceptable range.

Nodal Premature Beats and Nodal Escape Beats: Nodal (or junctional) premature beats and nodal escape beats are usually idiopathic, seen in otherwise normal newborn infants. They may be a sign of digitalis toxicity. Treatment is not indicated unless the cause is digitalis toxicity.

Nodal (or Junctional) Rhythm: Nodal rhythm may be seen in otherwise normal neonates, neonates with certain CHDs, and those with increased vagal tone (e.g., increased intracranial pressure, pharyngeal stimulation). No treatment is indicated if the patient is asymptomatic. Atropine or electrical pacing may be indicated if bradycardia is present.

Premature Ventricular Contractions: Many PVCs are idiopathic and are frequently seen in healthy newborns. Occasionally PVC is associated with CHDs, myocarditis, cardiomyopathy, or cardiac tumors, as well as hyperkalemia or asphyxia. Drugs such as catecholoamines, theophylline, and caffeine may be the cause. Rarely, a long QT syndrome (Jervell and Lange-Nielsen syndrome and Romano-Ward syndrome) may be responsible for the arrhythmia.

Occasional isolated uniform PVCs are usually benign. PVCs are most likely to be significant if (1) they are multiform, particularly couplets, (2) they are associated with underlying cardiac conditions, and (3) there are runs of PVCs.

Frequent PVCs require investigation, including an echo examination, and treatment. IV bolus lidocaine, followed by an IV drip of lidocaine, is a preferred approach. Other antiarrhythmic agents (e.g., phenytoin, propranolol) may be indicated.

Ventricular Tachycardia: Ventricular tachycardia is rare but more serious than any other arrhythmia. It may be associated with CHD, myocarditis, cardiomyopathy, or cardiac tumor, as well as hyperkalemia or asphyxia. Treatment consists of termination of the arrhythmia with lidocaine infusion or cardioversion, correction of the underlying cause when possible, and prevention of recurrence with antiarrhythmic agents (phenytoin, propranolol).

Atrioventricular Block

First-degree AV Block: Prolongation of the PR interval may be benign, although it may be a sign of digitalis toxicity, CHDs (e.g., ECD, ASD, and Ebstein anomaly), or metabolic abnormalities. No treatment is indicated except in digitalis toxicity.

Second-degree AV block: Myocarditis, cardiomyopathy, certain CHDs, postoperative state, and digitalis toxicity may cause second-degree AV block. Treatment should be directed at the underlying cause. Prophylactic pacemaker therapy may be indicated in Mobitz II or higher second-degree AV block.

Third-degree AV block: Complete heart block, or third-degree AV block, is due to a structural defect in the conduction system, usually above the bifurcation of the bundle of His (with narrow QRS complexes). About a third of cases are associated with CHDs. There is a frequent association of maternal lupus erythematosus or mixed connective tissue disease with congenital complete heart block in the offspring.

When complete heart block is associated with CHD, CHF usually results; pacemaker therapy is required. When complete heart block is not associated with CHD, pacemaker therapy is usually not necessary until childhood. There is 5% to 10% risk of sudden death in the first year of life. Indications for pacemaker therapy in the newborn are not completely established. However, pacemaker therapy is advised when some or all of the following risk factors are present: (1) heart rate persistently below 55 beats/min, (2) CHF resulting from associated CHDs, (3) significant cardiac anomalies, (4) escape ventricular beats, and (5) long QTc interval.

SPECIAL PROBLEMS

VII

I. CONGESTIVE HEART FAILURE

Etiology: Congestive heart failure (CHF) may result from congenital or acquired heart diseases with volume and/or pressure overload or from myocardial insufficiency.

1. CHD is the most common cause of CHF in children. The time of onset of CHF varies rather predictably with the type of the defect. Table 7-1 lists common CHDs according to the age at which CHF develops. Note that TOF and ASD do not cause CHF in children.

2. Acquired heart diseases can also cause CHF. Among valvular heart diseases, MR and AR are the two most common causes. CHF may be caused by myocardial dysfunction such as acute rheumatic fever, viral myocarditis, dilated cardiomyopathy, doxorubicin cardiomyopathy, endocardial fibroelastosis (EFE), and so on. Metabolic abnormalities (such as severe hypoxia and acidosis, hypoglycemia, and hypocalcemia in the newborn) can also cause it. The age at onset of CHF due to acquired heart disease is not as predictable as that of CHD.

3. Miscellaneous causes of CHF include such conditions as extreme tachycardia (e.g., SVT), complete heart block associated with structural heart defects, severe anemia, acute hypertension seen in acute postinfectious glomerulonephritis, brochopulmonary dysplasia seen in premature infants, and acute cor pulmonale due to acute airway obstruction (such as seen with large tonsils), and so on.

TABLE 7-1.

Causes of Congestive Heart Failure Due to Congenital Heart
Disease According to the Time of Occurrence

At birth	a. Hypoplastic left heart syndrome (HLHS)
	b. Volume overload lesions (e.g., severe TR or PR, large systemic AV fistula)
First week	a. Transposition of the great arteries (TGA)
	b. PDA in small premature infants
	c. HLHS (with more favorable anatomy)
	d. TAPVR, particularly those with pulmonary venous obstruction
	e. Critical AS or PS
	f. Others: Systemic AV fistula
1-4 weeks	a. COA (with associated anomalies)
	b. Critical AS
	c. Large L-R shunt lesions (e.g., VSD, PDA) in premature infants
	d. All other lesions listed above
4-6 weeks	a. Some L-R shunt lesions, such as ECD
6 weeks-4 months	a. Large VSD
	b. Large PDA
	c. Others: anomalous left coronary artery from the PA

Clinical Manifestations: No single test is specific for
CHF. The diagnosis of CHF relies on several sources of
clinical findings, including history, physical examination, and CXR film. Cardiomegaly on CXR films is
almost always present.

1. Poor feeding of recent onset, tachypnea, poor weight
gain, and cold sweat on the forehead suggest CHF in
infants. In older children shortness of breath, especially with activities, easy fatigability, puffy eyelids, or
swollen feet may be presenting complaints.

2. Physical findings can be divided by pathophysiologic
subgroups.

    a. Compensatory responses to impaired cardiac function

      1) Tachycardia, gallop rhythm, weak and thready pulse, and cardiomegaly.

      2) Signs of increased sympathetic discharges (growth failure, perspiration, and cold wet skin).

    b. Signs of pulmonary venous congestion (left-sided failure) include tachypnea, dyspnea on exertion (poor feeding in small infants), orthopnea in older children, and wheezing and pulmonary rales.

    c. Signs of systemic venous congestion (right-sided failure) include hepatomegaly and puffy eyelids. Distended neck veins and ankle edema are not seen in infants.

3. Cardiomegaly on CXR films is almost always present. The absence of cardiomegaly is a red flag against CHF.

4. The ECG may be helpful in determining the type of defects (but not helpful in deciding whether CHF is present).

5. Echo may confirm the presence of chamber enlargement or impaired LV function and determine the cause of CHF.

Management

1. General measures

    a. Cardiac chair and administration of oxygen (40% to 50%) with humidity may be used in infants with CHF.

    b. Sedation with morphine sulfate 0.1 to 0.2 mg/kg/dose q4h SC or phenobarbital 2 to 3 mg/kg/dose PO or IM q8h for 1 or 2 days is occasionally indicated.

    c. Salt restriction: A low-salt formula and severe fluid restriction are not indicated for infants; the use of diuretics has replaced these measures. In older children salt restriction (less than 0.5 g/day) and avoidance of salty snacks (chips, pretzels) and table salts are recommended.

    d. Daily weight measurement of hospitalized patients.

    e. Elimination or correction of predisposing factors (e.g., fever, anemia, infection).

    f. Treatment of underlying causes (hypertension, arrhythmias, or thyrotoxicosis).

2. Drug therapy: Three major classes of drugs are used in the treatment of CHF in children: inotropic agents, diuretics, and afterload-reducing agents. Every child with CHF should receive digitalis unless its use is contraindicated (e.g., hypertrophic cardiomyopathy, complete heart block, or cardiac tamponade). Diuretics are almost always used in conjunction with digitalis glycosides. Afterload-reducing agents have gained popularity in recent years.

    a. Diuretics: Patients with CHF often improve rapidly after a dose of a fast-acting diuretic, such as ethacrynic acid or furosemide, even before digitalization. Table 7-2 shows dosages of commonly available diuretic preparations. Side effects of diuretic

TABLE 7-2.

Diuretic Agents and Dosages

Preparation	Route	Dosage
Thiazide diuretics		
Chlorothiazide		
(Diuril)	Oral	20-40 mg/kg/day in two or three divided doses
Hydrochlorothiazide		
(HydroDiuril)	Oral	2-4 mg/kg/day in two or three divided doses
Loop diuretics		
Furosemide (Lasix)	IV	1 mg/kg/dose
	Oral	2-3 mg/kg/day in two or three divided doses
Ethacrynic acid		
(Edecrin)	IV	1 mg/kg/dose
	Oral	2-3 mg/kg/day in two or three divided doses
Aldosterone antagonists		
Spironolactone		
(Aldactone)	Oral	2-3 mg/kg/day in two or three divided doses

therapy include hypokalemia and hypochloremic alkalosis; both may increase the likelihood of digitalis toxicity.

b. Digitalis glycosides

1) Dosage of digoxin: The total digitalizing dose (TDD) and maintenance doses of digoxin by oral (and IV) routes are shown in Table 7-3. (The dosage of digitoxin appears in Chapter 9, Cardiovascular Drug Dosage.) The dosage may be higher in treating SVT, in which the goal of treatment is to delay AV conduction. The maintenance dose, not the loading dose, is closely related to the serum digoxin level.

2) The following is a suggested step-by-step method of digitalization:

a) Obtain a baseline ECG with a rhythm strip (for rhythm and the PR interval) and serum electrolytes.

b) Give one half TDD *stat* followed by one fourth and the final one fourth of the TDD at 6 to 8 hour intervals.

c) Start the maintenance dose 12 hours after the final TDD.

TABLE 7-3.

Oral Digoxin Dosage for Congestive Heart Failure

	TDD* (µg/kg)	Maintenance*† (µg/kg/day)
Prematures	20	5
Newborns	30	8
Under 2 yr	40-50	10-12
Over 2 yr	30-40	8-10

TDD, total digitalizing dose.
*IV dose is 75% of the oral dose.
†Maintenance dose is 25% of the TDD in 2 divided doses.
From Park MK: *The use of digoxin in infants and children with specific emphasis on dosage.* J. Pediatr *108:871-877, 1986.*

TABLE 7-4.

Factors That May Predispose to Digitalis Toxicity

High serum digoxin level
    High-dose requirement, as in treatment of certain arrhythmias
    Decreased renal excretion (premature infants, renal disease)
    Hypothyroidism
    Drug interaction (e.g., quinidine, verapamil, amiodarone)
Increased sensitivity of myocardium (without high serum digoxin
    level)
    Status of myocardium (myocardial ischemia, rheumatic or viral
      myocarditis)
    Systemic changes (electrolytes [↓K, ↑Ca], hypoxia, alkalosis)
    Catecholamines
    Immediate postoperative period after heart surgery under CPB

      d) Obtain ECGs to check on possible signs of
         digitalis toxicity before the final TDD dose
         or the first maintenance dose.
    3) Monitoring for digitalis toxicity by ECG: With
      the relatively low dosage recommended in Table
      7-3, digitalis toxicity is unlikely unless there are
      predisposing factors for the toxicity (Table 7-4).
      During the first 3 to 5 days after digitalization,
      during which time the pharmacokinetic steady
      state is not reached, detection of digitalis tox-
      icity is best accomplished by monitoring with
      ECGs, not by serum digoxin levels. Table 7-5
      lists ECG signs of digitalis effects and toxicity. In
      general, the digitalis effect is confined to *ven-*
      tricular repolarization, whereas toxicity involves
      disturbances in the *formation and conduction*
      of the impulse. A sound rule is to assume that any
      arrhythmia or conduction disturbance occur-
      ring with digitalis is caused by digitalis until
      proven otherwise.
    4) Serum digoxin levels: Therapeutic ranges of se-
      rum digoxin levels for treating CHF are 0.8 to 2
      ng/ml. Levels obtained during the first 3 to 5
      days after digitalization tend to be higher than

TABLE 7-5.

ECG Changes Associated with Digitalis

Effects
  Shortening of QTc is the earliest sign of digitalis effect.
  Sagging ST segment and diminished amplitude of T wave
    (T vector does not change).
  Slowing of heart rate.
Toxicity
  Prolongation of PR interval.
    Some normal children have prolonged PR interval, making
    it mandatory to obtain a baseline ECG. May progress to
    advanced AV block.
  Profound sinus bradycardia or sinoatrial block.
  Supraventricular arrhythmias (atrial or nodal ectopic beats and
    tachycardias), particularly if accompanied by AV block, are
    more common than ventricular arrhythmias in children.
  Ventricular arrhythmias (such as ventricular bigeminy or tri-
    geminy) are extremely rare in children, although common in
    adults with digitalis toxicity. Isolated PVCs are not uncommon
    in children as a sign of toxicity.

those obtained when the pharmacokinetic
steady state is reached (5 to 8 days). Serum
digoxin levels should be drawn at least 6 hours
after the last dose or just before a scheduled
dose; samples obtained before 6 hours after the
last dose will give a falsely elevated level. Determining serum digoxin levels often and using
those levels for therapeutic goals are neither
justified nor practical; occasional determination
of the level is adequate. A serum digoxin level
greater than 2 ng/ml is likely associated with
toxicity if the clinical findings suggest digitalis
toxicity. Patients with any of the conditions
listed in Table 7-4 are likely to develop toxicity.
5) Endogenous digoxin-like substance (EDLS):
    EDLS is found in some normal full term and
    preterm newborn infants who are not even re-
    ceiving digoxin. EDLS is also found in some
    adults with various conditions such as renal, he-

patic, or heart failure; pregnancy; hypertension; and volume expansion or electrolyte imbalance as well as after treadmill exercise. EDLS was shown to have digitalis-like actions, including inhibition of the Na-K-ATPase and demonstrable cardiotonic effects. Recently it has been shown that EDLS is probably ouabain, a cardiac glycoside. The potency of the inotropic effect of ouabain is similar to that of digoxin. Therefore it does not appear justified to allow a high serum digoxin level or to disregard the digoxin level in the newborn on account of a possible contamination of digoxin levels by EDLS.

6) Other inotropic agents: In infants in severe CHF with distress, patients with renal dysfunction (such as seen in symptomatic infants with COA) or in those with postoperative cardiac failure, rapidly acting catecholamines with short duration of action are preferable to digoxin. Suggested dosages of catecholamines for IV drips are shown in Table 7-6.

7) Afterload-reducing agents: Reducing the afterload tends to augment the stroke volume without changes in the contractile state of the heart and therefore without increasing myocardial oxygen consumption. These agents are usually used in conjunction with digitalis glycosides and diuretics. In addition to myocardial dysfunction, patients with CHF from large L-R shunts (such as VSD, AV canal, PDA) have been shown to benefit from hydralazine and captopril.

Depending on the site of action, afterload-reducing agents are divided into three groups: arteriolar vasodilators (hydralazine), venodilators (nitroglycerin, isosorbide dinitrate), and mixed, or balanced vasodilators (ACE inhibitors [such as captopril and enalapril], nitroprusside, and prazosin). Dosages of vasodilator agents are presented in Table 7-7.

TABLE 7-6.

Suggested Starting Dosages of Catecholamines

Drug	Route and Dosage	Side Effects
Epinephrine (Adrenalin)	IV 0.1-1 µg/kg/min	Hypertension, arrhythmias
Isoproterenol (Isuprel)	IV 0.1-0.5 µg/kg/min	Peripheral and pulmonary vasodilation
Dobutamine (Dobutrex)	IV 5-8 µg/kg/min	Little tachycardia and vasodilation, arrhythmias
Dopamine (Intropin)	IV 5-10 µg/kg/min	Tachycardia, arrhythmias, hypertension or hypotension
		Dose-related cardiovascular effects of dopamine (µg/kg/min)
		Renal vasodilation 2-5
		Inotropic 5-8
		Tachycardia >8
		Mild vasoconstrict. >10
		Vasoconstriction 15-20

3. Surgical management: If medical treatment is not successful in improving CHF in infants with CHDs within a few weeks to months, specific palliative or corrective cardiac surgery should be performed.

II. CHEST PAIN

Chest pain is a common complaint heard from children in the office or emergency room. Although chest pain does not indicate serious disease of the heart or other systems in most children, chest pain means "heart disease" to most of these children and their parents. Physicians should be aware of the differential diagnosis of chest pain in children and should make every effort to find a specific cause before reassuring the child and the parents. Making a referral to a cardiologist is not always a good idea; it may actually increase the family's concern.

TABLE 7-7.
Dosages of Vasodilators

Drug	Route and Dosage	Comments
Hydralazine (Apresoline)	IV 1.5 µg/kg/min, or 0.1-0.2 mg/kg/dose, q4-6h; max 2 mg/kg q6h PO 0.75-3 mg/kg/day in two to four doses; max 200 mg/day	May cause tachycardia; may use with pro-pranolol; gastrointestinal symptoms, neutropenia, lupuslike syndrome.
Nitroglycerin	IV 0.5-2 µg/kg/min; max 6 µg/kg/min	Start with a small dose and titrate effects.
Captopril (Capoten)	PO NB: 0.1-0.4 mg/kg/dose q.d.-q.i.d. Infants 0.5-6 mg/kg/day in 1 to 4 doses Child 12.5 mg/dose q.d.-b.i.d.	Hypotension, dizziness; may cause neu-tropenia, proteinuria; reduce dose in patients with impaired renal function.
Enalapril (Vasotec)	PO 0.1 mg/kg q.d.-b.i.d.	May develop hypotension, dizziness, or syncope.
Nitroprusside (Nipride)	IV 0.5-8 µg/kg/min	May cause thiocyanate or cyanide toxicity (e.g., fatigue, nausea, disorientation); hepatic dysfunction, light sensitivity
Prazosin (Minipress)	PO First dose: 5 µg/kg Increase to 25-150 µg/kg/day in four doses	Fewer side effects than hydralazine; ortho-static hypotension; tachyphylaxis may develop

Etiology: Causes of chest pain in children are listed in Table 7-8. The three most common, accounting for 45% to 65%, are costochondritis, chest wall pathology (trauma, muscle strain), and respiratory diseases, especially those associated with coughing (Table 7-9). Cardiac diseases rarely cause chest pain in children (0 to 4%). No cause is found in up to 40% of the patients even after moderately extensive studies. Psychologic cause of chest pain is found in 5% to 10% of patients, but this diagnosis should not be assigned without thorough history taking and follow-up evaluation.

Clinical Manifestations: These are the pertinent clinical features of the three most common causes of chest pain in children:

1. Costochondritis is characterized by mild to moderate anterior chest pain, usually unilateral but occasionally bilateral. The pain may be preceded by exercise or an upper respiratory infection, and physical activity or a specific position may bring on the pain. The pain may radiate to the remainder of the chest, back, and abdomen; it may be exaggerated by breathing, and it may persist for several months. Physical examination is diagnostic; one finds a reproducible tenderness on palpation over the chondrosternal and/or costochondral junctions. It is a benign condition.

2. Musculoskeletal chest pain is caused by strains of the pectoral, the shoulder, or the back muscles after exercise or by trauma to the chest wall from sports, fights or accidents. History of vigorous exercise, weight lifting, or direct trauma to the chest and tenderness of the chest wall or muscles are clear evidence of muscle strain or trauma.

3. Respiratory chest pain may result from overused chest wall muscles or pleural irritation. A history of severe cough with tenderness of intercostal or abdominal muscles is usually present. Rales, wheezing, tachypnea, retraction, or fever on examination suggests respiratory chest pain. Pleural effusion may cause pain that is worsened by deep inspiration. CXR films

TABLE 7-8.

Causes of Chest Pain in Children

Noncardiac Causes

  Thoracic cage
    Costochondritis
    Trauma or muscle strain
    Abnormalities of rib cage or thoracic spine
    Breast tenderness (mastalgia)
  Respiratory system
    Severe cough or bronchitis
    Pleural effusion
    Lobar pneumonia
    Exercise-induced asthma
    Spontaneous pneumothorax or pneumomediastinum
  Gastrointestinal system
  Psychogenic origins
    Hyperventilation
    Conversion symptoms
    Somatization disorder
    Depression
  Miscellaneous origins
    Texidor's twinge
    Herpes zoster
    Pleurododynia

Cardiac Causes

  Ischemic ventricular dysfunction
    Structural abnormalities of heart (Severe AS or PS, HOCM,
      Eisenmenger syndrome)
    Mitral valve prolapse
    Coronary artery abnormalities (old Kawasaki, congenital
      anomaly, coronary heart disease, hypertension, sickle cell
      disease)
    Cocaine (drug abuse)
    Aortic dissection and aortic aneurysm (Turner, Marfan, or
      Noonan syndrome)
  Inflammation
    Pericarditis (viral, bacterial, or rheumatic)
    Postpericardiotomy syndrome
    Myocarditis, acute or chronic
    Kawasaki disease
  Arrhythmias (with palpitation)
    Supraventricular tachycardia
    Frequent PVCs or ventricular tachycardia (?)

TABLE 7-9.

Incidence of Causes of Chest Pain in Children

Cause	Incidence
Idiopathic	12-45%
Costochondritis	9-22
Musculoskeletal trauma	21
Cough, asthma, pneumonia	15-21
Psychogenic cause	5-9
Gastrointestinal system	4-7
Cardiac disorder	0-4
Sickle cell crisis	2
Miscellaneous	9-21

may confirm the diagnosis of pleural effusion, pneumonia, or pneumothorax. Asthma causes chest pain on exertion in some children, but it may not be suspected until stress tests reveal exercise-induced asthma.

Diagnostic Approach: A three-step approach is recommended (Table 7-10). The first step should be directed toward detecting the three most common causes of chest pain, i.e., costochondritis, musculoskeletal causes, and respiratory diseases, which together account for 45% to 65% of chest pain in children. A thorough history and physical examination are all that are required to make the diagnosis of these three conditions. The second step is to check for cardiac causes, with physical examination of the cardiovascular system, CXR film, and an ECG. If no cardiac cause is found, the pain is probably due to either other systemic disease, including psychogenic or idiopathic causes (the third stage).

Step 1: The initial history should be directed at finding out the nature of the pain, associated symptoms, and concurrent or precipitating events that may help in clarifying the noncardiac or cardiac origin of the pain. Past and family histories are also important in determining cardiac or noncardiac causes of the pain. The single most important

TABLE 7-10.

Three-Step Approach to Chest Pain

Step 1: The three most common causes of chest pain in children (45%-65%) (costochondritis, musculoskeletal causes, and respiratory diseases) are sought by history and physical examination.

Step 2: Cardiac causes (0%-4%) of chest pain are sought. CXR film and ECG are needed in addition to history and careful cardiac examination (see Table 7-11 for differential diagnosis)

Step 3: Other systemic disease, including psychogenic and idiopathic causes (15%-45%) are likely. Follow-up may clarify the cause.

---

feature of cardiac causes of chest pain is its precipitation by exertion and the quality of pain, which is described as a pressure sensation or squeezing, not a sharp pain. A screen for cocaine may be worthwhile in adolescents who present with acute, severe chest pain and distress with an unclear cause. The following are some questions that should be asked.

a. History of present illness
   1) What seems to bring on the pain—(exercise, eating, trauma, emotional stress)? Do you get the same type of pain while you watch TV or sitting in class?
   2) What is the pain like—(sharp, pressure sensation, squeezing nature?).
   3) Location (specific point, localized or diffuse), severity, radiation, and duration (seconds, minutes).
   4) Does the pain get worse with deep breathing? (If so, it may be due to pleural irritation or chest wall pathology.) Or does the pain improve with certain body positions (seen sometimes with pericarditis)?
   5) How often and for how long have you had similar pain?
   6) Have you been hurt while playing or have you used your arms excessively for any reason?

       7) Do you have any associated symptoms, such as cough, fever, syncope, dizziness or palpitation?

       8) Are you on any medications, including birth control pills? Have you been using drugs (cocaine) or cigarettes?

       9) What treatments for the pain have already been tried?

  b. Past and family history

       1) Are there any known medical conditions (e.g., congenital or acquired heart disease, cardiac surgery, infection, asthma)?

       2) Has there been recent heart disease, chest pain, or cardiac death in the family?

       3) Does any disease run in the family?

       4) What is the patient or family member concerned about?

4. Physical examination should also be directed at finding causes based on the history.

  a. Is the child in severe distress from pain, in emotional stress, or hyperventilating?

  b. Is there bruising elsewhere on the body (this may imply invisible chest trauma)?

  c. The chest should be carefully inspected for trauma or asymmetry. The chest wall should be palpated for signs of tenderness or subcutaneous air. Special attention should be paid to the possibility of costochondritis by palpating each one of the costochondral and chondrosternal junctions.

  d. The heart and lungs should be auscultated for arrhythmias, heart murmurs, rubs, muffled heart sounds, gallop rhythm, rales, wheezes, or decreased breath sounds.

  e. The abdomen should be carefully examined because it may be the source of referred pain to the chest.

    Step 2: Examination for cardiac causes of chest pain. If none of the three common causes or other identifiable causes of chest pain is found, attention should be directed to each of the cardiac causes of

TABLE 7-11.

Important Clinical Findings of Cardiac Causes of Chest Pain

Conditions	History	Physical Examination	ECG	CXR Film
Severe AS	CHD (+)	Loud (>grade 3/6) systolic ejection murmur at URSB with radiation to the neck	LVH with or without strain	Prominent ascending aorta and aortic knob
Severe PS	CHD (+)	Loud (grade >3/6) systolic ejection murmur at ULSB	RVH with or without strain	Prominent MPA segment
HOCM	FH (+) in 33% of cases	Variable heart murmurs; brisk brachial pulses (±)	LVH Deep Q/small R or QS pattern in LPLs	Mild cardiomegaly with globular heart
MVP	Positive FH (±)	Midsystolic click with or without late systolic murmur; thin body build; thoracic skeletal anomalies (80%)	Inverted T waves in aVF (±)	Normal heart size; straight back (±); narrow AP diameter (±)
Eisenmenger syndrome	CHD (+)	Cyanosis or clubbing; RV impulse; loud and single S2; soft or no heart murmur	RVH	Markedly prominent MPA with normal heart size
Anomalous origin of left coronary artery	Symptomatic in early infancy, with recurrent episodes of distress	Soft or no heart murmur	MI, anterolateral	Moderate to marked cardiomegaly

Sequelae of Kawasaki or other coronary artery disease	Kawasaki disease (±); typical exercise-related anginal pain	Usually normal; continuous murmur in coronary fistula	ST-segment elevation (±); old MI pattern (±)	May be normal or mild cardiomegaly
Cocaine abuse	Substance abuse (±)	Hypertension; nonspecific heart murmur (±)	ST segment elevation (±)	May be normal in acute cases
Pericarditis, myocarditis	URI (±); sharp chest pain	Friction rub; muffled heart sounds; nonspecific heart murmur (±)	Low QRS voltages; ST segment shift; arrhythmias (±)	Cardiomegaly of varying degree
Postpericardiotomy syndrome	Recent heart surgery; sharp pain; dyspnea	Muffled heart sounds (±); friction rub	Persistent ST-segment elevation	Cardiomegaly of varying degree
Arrhythmias (+palpitation)	WPW (±); FH of long QT syndrome	May be normal; irregular rhythm (±)	Arrhythmias (±); WPW syndrome (±); long QTc (>0.46 sec)	Normal

AP, anteroposterior; AS, aortic stenosis; CHD, congenital heart disease; FH, family history; HOCM, hypertrophic obstructive cardiomyopathy; LVH, left ventricular hypertrophy; LPLs, left precordial leads; MI, myocardial infarction; MPA, main pulmonary artery; MVP, mitral valve prolapse; PS, pulmonary stenosis; RV, right ventricular; RVH, right ventricular hypertrophy; ULSB, upper left sternal border; URI, upper respiratory infection; URSB, upper right sternal border; WPW, Wolff-Parkinson-White syndrome.

chest pain (Table 7-8). Most patients with cardiac causes of chest pain have a history of cardiac problems and the diagnosis.

Even though cardiac causes are not high on the differential diagnosis, CXR film and an ECG are usually indicated at this stage. CXR film should be evaluated for pulmonary pathology, cardiac size and silhouette, and pulmonary vascularity. The ECG should be interpreted with special attention to arrhythmias, hypertrophy, conduction disturbances, including WPW syndrome, abnormal T waves and Q waves, and the QT interval. Table 7-11 summarizes important history, physical findings, and abnormalities of CXR film and ECG for cardiac causes of chest pain.

Step 3: If the family history is negative for hereditary heart disease, if the history is negative for heart disease and Kawasaki disease, if cardiac examination is unremarkable, and if the ECG and CXR film are normal, cardiac causes of chest pain are practically ruled out. The patient is likely to have either idiopathic or psychogenic pain or an abnormality of another system. At this point one can reassure the patient and family of a probable benign nature of the chest pain. Simple follow-up of these patients may clarify the cause of the pain.

Management: When a specific cause of chest pain is identified, treatment is directed at correcting or improving the cause.

1. Costochondritis can be treated by reassurance and occasionally by acetaminophen or nonsteroidal antiinflammatory agents.

2. Most musculoskeletal and nonorganic causes of chest pain can be treated with local rest, acetaminophen, or nonsteroidal antiinflammatory agents.

3. If a respiratory cause is found, treatment is directed to it.

4. The following are some of the indications for a referral of a child with chest pain for cardiac evaluation.

a. Chest pain suggesting angina and abnormal findings in cardiac examination or abnormalities in CXR film or the ECG.

b. Family history of cardiomyopathy, long QT syndrome, or other hereditary disease with which cardiac abnormalities are commonly associated.

c. A high level of anxiety of the family and/or the patient or chronic, recurring pain.

5. The correct therapy of acute cocaine toxicity is not well established. Calcium channel blockers (nifedipine, nitrendipine), β-adrenergic blockers, nitrates, and thrombolytic agents have resulted in varying levels of success. The use of β-blockers is controversial; they may worsen coronary blood flow.

III. SYNCOPE

Etiology: Syncope is loss or near loss of consciousness, frequently with loss of muscle tone, for less than 1 min. It may be due to circulatory, metabolic, or neuropsychologic causes. Normal function of the brain depends on a constant supply of oxygen and glucose. Significant alterations in their supply may result in such transient faintness. Table 7-12 lists possible causes of syncope.

Clinical Manifestations: A description of some important or common causes of syncope follows; history is important in the differential diagnosis.

1. Vasovagal syncope (vasodepressor, neurocardiogenic, or common syncope) is the most common noncardiac type. It is characterized by a few seconds to a minute of a prodrome of dizziness, pallor, palpitation, diaphoresis, nausea, light-headedness, and hyperventilation followed by loss of consciousness and muscle tone. The patient falls, usually without injury, and the unconsciousness does not last more than a minute, with gradual awakening. It usually occurs in association with anxiety or fright, pain, blood drawing (or the sight of blood), fasting, heat and humidity, a crowded place, or prolonged motionless standing.

TABLE 7-12.

Etiologic Classification of Syncope

Circulatory Causes
  Extracardiac causes
    Common faint or vasovagal syncope
    Orthostatic hypotension
    Failure of venous return (e.g., increased intrathoracic pressure, decreased venous return, hypovolemia)
    Cerebrovascular occlusive disease
  Intracardiac causes
    Severe obstructive disease (e.g., AS, PS, HOCM, pulmonary hypertension)
    Myocardial dysfunction (e.g., myocardial ischemia or infarction, Kawasaki disease, coronary artery anomalies)
    Arrhythmias (extreme tachycardia or bradycardia, long QT syndrome)

Metabolic Causes
  Hypoglycemia
  Hyperventilation syndrome
  Hypoxia

Neuropsychiatric Causes
  Epilepsy
  Brain tumor
  Migraine
  Hysteria or nonconvulsive seizures

The diagnosis is made by typical history and by exclusion of other causes.

2. Orthostatic hypotension is characterized by absent or inadequate response of normal adrenergic vasoconstriction of arterioles and veins in the upright position, resulting in hypotension without a reflex increase in heart rate. In contrast to the prodrome of vasovagal syncope, patients with orthostatic hypotension are only light-headed. There may be a history of prolonged bed rest, prolonged standing, dehydration, or medications (such as calcium channel blockers, antihypertensive drugs, vasodilators, phenothiazines, or diuretics).

3. Hyperventilation spells produce hypocapnia, resulting in an intense cerebral vasoconstriction. A typical spell usually begins with an apprehensive feeling with deep sighing respirations that the patient rarely notices. The patient often has abdominal discomfort, palpitations, light-headedness, and rarely loss of consciousness.

4. Epilepsy may be accompanied by incontinence, marked confusion in the postictal state, and an abnormal EEG. The patient is rigid rather than limp and may have sustained an injury. The patient does not have the early symptoms of syncope (dizziness, pallor, palpitation, diaphoresis). The duration of unconsciousness is longer than is typical of syncope (less than 1 minute).

5. Hypoglycemia has characteristics similar to those of syncope, such as pallor, perspiration, abdominal discomfort, light-headedness, confusion, unconsciousness, and possible subsequent seizures. However, hypoglycemic attacks differ from syncope in that the onset and recovery are more gradual, they do not occur during or shortly after meals, and the presyncopal symptoms do not improve when the patient is supine.

6. Hysteria with syncope, which is not associated with injury, occurs only in the presence of an audience. A teenager may be able to give an accurate presyncopal history but does not have the pallor and hypotension that characterize true syncope. The attacks may last longer (up to an hour) than a brief syncopal spell. Episodes usually occur in an emotionally charged setting and are rare in patients less than age 10.

7. Cardiac syncope may be due to structural heart disease or secondary to arrhythmias. A cardiac cause is suggested by syncope even while recumbent, syncope provoked by exercise, chest pain associated with syncope, history of heart disease, and family history of sudden death. Cardiac causes of syncope are obstructive lesions, coronary insufficiency, and arrhythmias, including long QT syndrome. Either extreme tachy-

cardia or bradycardia can decrease cardiac output
and lower the cerebral blood flow below the critical
level, causing syncope.

Diagnostic Approach

1. History: A thorough and accurate history is more important than a physical examination; it is essential in
   deciding a cost-effective diagnostic work-up for each
   individual patient. History taking should be directed
   at three common noncardiac causes of syncope: vasovagal attack (the most common), orthostatic hypotension, and hyperventilation. Exercise-related
   syncope may be caused by arrhythmias, which need
   special evaluation.
   a. Precipitating factors—suddenness of onset, pro-
      gression, duration, presyncopal symptoms, dura-
      tion of any unconsciousness, and the recovery
      period—are all important.
   b. Accompanying signs and symptoms, such as pallor,
      diaphoresis, palpitation, and nausea, are also im-
      portant.
   c. Associated diseases and sequelae, medications,
      medical history, recent illness, metabolic disease,
      social interactions, and family history should also
      be obtained.
2. Physical examination
   a. In vasovagal syncope, since the patient presents af-
      ter the event, the physical examination is usually
      normal. History taking is very important.
   b. If orthostatic hypotension is suspected, the pulse
      rate and blood pressure are each measured with
      the patient supine and standing (after standing for
      5 to 10 minutes). A 10 to 15 mm Hg drop in sys-
      tolic pressure is abnormal, especially if the heart
      rate does not compensate by increasing.
   c. If hyperventilation syncope is suspected, the pa-
      tient may be made to hyperventilate to reproduce
      the phenomenon.
3. Laboratory studies
   a. Further investigation is required if the faint is exer-
      cise induced or preceded by chest pain, if there is

evidence of seizure activity or loss of bowel or bladder control, if the faint is atypical of vasovagal syncope, if the syncope recurs more than two or three times, if physical examination suggests a cardiovascular abnormality, or if there is a family history of unexplained death.

b. Initial laboratory studies may include ECG, CXR film, serum electrolytes, fasting blood glucose, and an EEG.

4. Further studies will probably be directed by the cardiology or neurology service and may include some or all of the following: echocardiography and color flow Doppler studies, 24-hour ambulatory ECG monitoring, treadmill exercise test for cardiovascular abnormalities, and a CT scan of the brain for neurologic evaluation. Head-up tilt test, with or without isoproterenol infusion, has been recommended by some for evaluation of syncope of unknown origin, but it has not been well standardized, and its specificity and reproducibility are questionable.

Treatment: When the cause is identified, the treatment is directed at the cause.

1. For vasovagal syncope the following may be tried:
   a. Placing the patient in a supine position may be all that is indicated. If the patient feels the prodrome for a faint, it can be aborted by lying and raising the feet.
   b. Varying levels of success in preventing syncope have been reported with the use of fluorocortisone; metoprolol 1.5 mg/kg/day PO in two or three doses for children; disopyramide; oral pseudoephedrine 60 mg b.i.d. PO for older children and adolescents, or transdermal scopolamine.
   c. An implanted pacemaker may maintain the heart rate but not prevent blood pressure from dropping, resulting in syncope.

2. For orthostatic hypotension elastic stockings, high-salt diet, sympathomimetic amines, and corticosteroids have been used with varying degrees of success. The patient should be told to get up slowly.

IV. LONG QT SYNDROME

The patient with a long QT syndrome may present with syncope or seizures. This syndrome is characterized by prolongation of the QT interval on the ECG and is accompanied by a high incidence of lethal ventricular arrhythmias. There are three groups of patients in this syndrome:

1. Jervell and Lange-Nielsen syndrome is characterized by a long QT interval on the ECG, congenital deafness, syncopal spells, and history of sudden death in the family. This syndrome is transmitted as an autosomal recessive pattern.

2. Romano-Ward syndrome has all the features of Jervell and Lange-Nielsen syndrome except deafness. This syndrome transmits in an autosomal dominant mode.

3. A significant number of affected individuals with normal hearing appear to represent sporadic cases, with negative family history of the syndrome.

Clinical Manifestations

1. The family history is positive in about 60% and deafness is present in 5% of patients with long QT syndrome. Presenting symptoms may be syncope, seizure, cardiac arrest, or palpitation. The majority of these symptoms occur during exercise and/or with emotion and are usually manifested by the end of the second decade of life.

2. The ECG shows a prolonged QT interval with a corrected QT (QTc) interval greater than 0.44 sec. In addition, bradycardia, second-degree AV block, multiform PVCs, monomorphic or polymorphic ventricular tachycardia, and abnormal T wave morphology (bifid, diphasic, or notched) are common; all of these are considered to be risk factors for sudden death.

3. A treadmill exercise test produces highly significant prolongation of the QTc interval in response to exercise, with the maximal prolongation present after 2 min of recovery. Ventricular arrhythmias develop during the test (in up to 30% of the patients).

Diagnosis: The high risk of sudden death in untreated patients requires a correct diagnosis so that proper and effective treatment can be instituted. On the other hand, the diagnosis of this disease with a poor prognosis should not be made lightly, as it may imply a lifelong commitment to treatment.

The Pediatric Electrophysiology Society (Garson, 1993) used the following two criteria:

1. A QTc interval of at least 0.44 sec in the absence of other underlying causes such as prematurity, electrolyte disturbance, or central nervous system abnormality.

2. A family history of long QT syndrome *plus* unexplained syncope, seizure, or cardiac arrest associated with typical inciting events such as exercise or emotion, even if the QTc interval is normal (less than 0.44 sec). (The QTc can vary over time.)

The first criterion is debatable, since as many as 1% to 4% of normal children have a QTc above 0.46 sec. Such an inclusion becomes important in light of the possibility of lifelong prophylactic treatment of asymptomatic children. In children with a borderline prolongation of the QTc interval, a repeat ECG and a treadmill test or a Holter monitoring may be worthwhile. These tests may show a more convincing prolongation of the QTc interval.

Lead II is the preferred lead to measure the QT interval. The QTc interval is calculated by using Bazette's formula (see Chapter 1). The QTc interval represents the QT interval normalized for a heart rate of 60 beats/min. The longest QTc interval is the one that follows the shortest RR interval. The QTc is longer during sleep, and therefore Holter monitoring may show the QTc interval 0.05 sec longer than the interval on a standard ECG.

Treatment

1. Long QT syndrome is a serious disease that can result in sudden death, and treatment is at best only partially effective. Risk factors should be considered in the treatment plan.

    a. Risk factors for sudden death include bradycardia for age (sinus bradycardia, junctional escape rhythm, or second-degree AV block), extremely long QTc (above 0.55 sec), symptoms at presenta-

tion (syncope, seizure, cardiac arrest), youth at
presentation (under 1 month), and documented
torsade de pointes or ventricular fibrillation.
   b. T wave alternation (major changes in T wave morphology) is a relative risk factor.
   c. Noncompliance with medication is an important
risk factor for sudden death.
   d. Low risk is found for children with a normal QTc
interval, no symptoms, and only a positive family
history.
2. The three major treatment modalities for the syndrome are β-adrenergic blockers, left cardiac sympathetic denervation, and demand cardiac pacemaker.
   a. β-Blockers: The present therapy of choice is treatment with β-blockers (propranolol, atenolol, metoprolol). There is consensus that all symptomatic
children with the long QT syndrome should be
treated with propranolol or another β-blocker.
Moderate doses may be better than larger ones because they lessen the trend toward bradycardia, a
known risk factor for sudden death, especially in
patients with a sinus or AV nodal disorder. Even
with treatment with β-blockers, sudden death can
occur: over 80% of sudden deaths occurred while
the patients were on medications. Some deaths
were due to noncompliance.
      Whether to treat asymptomatic children with a
QTc interval 0.44 sec or slightly longer and a
positive family history of the long QT syndrome is
controversial. Instead of receiving treatment with
β-blockers, these children may be followed closely
for the development of prolongation of the QTc
interval or symptoms. If these occur, treatment
is clearly indicated.
   b. Left cardiac sympathetic denervation: For patients
who continue to have syncope or ventricular tachycardia, left cardiac sympathetic denervation, preferably a high thoracic left sympathectomy, may
prove effective. Other denervation surgeries, such
as left stellectomy and left cervicothoracic sympa-

thectomy, almost always result in Horner syndrome and often provide inadequate cardiac sympathetic denervation. Sudden death still occurs (8%); the 5-year survival rate is 94%.

c. Demand cardiac pacemaker: Implantation of pacemaker and/or defibrillator may be considered for high risk patients, especially those with a QTc above 0.6 sec. However, it does not provide complete protection from sudden death (16%). Patients should be kept on β-blockers.

V. SYSTEMIC HYPERTENSION

Definition

1. A child has *high normal BP* when the average systolic and/or diastolic BP is between the ninetieth and ninety-fifth percentile for age. *Hypertension* is present when systolic and/or diastolic BP is greater than the ninety-fifth percentile for age on at least on three occasions.

2. The World Health Organization (WHO) defines adult borderline hypertension as BP of 140/90 to 150/95; in hypertension the BP is 160/95 or higher.

Etiology: Causes of hypertension are listed in Table 7-13. Primary (or essential) hypertension is rare before age 10. Over 90% of secondary hypertension in children is caused by three conditions: renal parenchymal disease, renal artery disease, and COA. In general, the younger the child and the more severe the hypertension, the more likely one is to identify an underlying cause.

Diagnosis and Work-Up: Careful evaluation of history, physical findings, and simple laboratory tests usually points to the cause of hypertension.

1. History
   a. Past and present history
      1) Neonatal: use of umbilical artery catheters.
      2) Cardiovascular: COA or surgery for it. History of palpitation, headache, and excessive sweating (suggest excessive catecholamines).

TABLE 7-13.

Causes of Hypertension

Primary (or essential) hypertension—causes not known
Secondary hypertension
  Renal
    Renal parenchymal disease: glomerulonephritis, pyelone-
      phritis, polycystic or dysplastic kidneys, hydronephrosis,
      hemolytic uremic syndrome, collagen disease (periarteritis,
      lupus), renal damage from nephrotoxic medications, trauma,
      or radiation.
    Renovascular diseases: renal artery stenosis, polyarteritis,
      renal artery or vein thrombosis.
  Cardiovascular: COA.
  Endocrine.
  Hyperthyroidism.
    Excessive catecholamines: pheochromocytoma, neuro-
      blastoma.
    Adrenal dysfunction: congenital adrenal hyperplasia, Cush-
      ing's syndrome, hyperaldosteronism (primary or secondary),
      hyperparathyroidism.
  Neurogenic: increased intracranial pressure, poliomyelitis,
    Guillain-Barré syndrome, dysautonomia.
  Drugs and chemicals: sympathomimetic drugs (nose drops,
    cough medications, cold preparations), amphetamines,
    steroids, oral contraceptives, heavy metal (mercury, lead)
    poisoning, cocaine, acute or chronic use.
  Miscellaneous: hypervolemia and hypernatremia, Stevens-
    Johnson syndrome, bronchopulmonary dysplasia (newborn).

---

    3) Renal: obstructive uropathies, urinary tract in-
       fection, radiation, trauma, or surgery to the
       kidney area.
    4) Endocrine: weakness and muscle cramp (hyper-
       aldosteronism).
    5) Medications: corticosteroids, amphetamines, an-
       tiasthmatic drugs, cold medications, oral contra-
       ceptives, nephrotoxic antibiotics.
    6) Habits: smoking
  b. Family
    1) Essential hypertension, atherosclerotic heart
       disease, and stroke.

2) Familial or hereditary renal disease (polycystic kidney, cystinuria, familial nephritis).

2. Physical examination
   a. Accurate measurement of blood pressure is essential (see Chapter 1 for method and normative BP levels).
   b. Complete physical examination should be performed with emphasis on delayed growth (renal disease), bounding peripheral pulse (PDA or AR), weak or absent femoral pulses (COA), abdominal bruits (renovascular disorder), and tenderness of the kidney (renal infection).

3. Laboratory tests
   Table 7-14 summarizes the routine and specialized tests used in identifying the cause of secondary hypertension.
   a. Initial laboratory tests are directed at detecting renal parenchymal disease, renovascular disease, and COA: urinalysis, urine culture, serum electrolytes, BUN, or creatinine, uric acid, ECG, CXR films, and possibly echo.
   b. Children under age 10 with sustained hypertension require extensive evaluation, since identifiable and possibly curable causes are likely to be found.
   c. Adolescents with mild hypertension and family history of essential hypertension are likely to have essential hypertension, and extensive studies are not indicated.

Management

1. Essential hypertension
   a. Nonpharmacologic intervention initially: weight reduction, low-salt (and potassium-rich) diet, physical fitness, and avoidance of smoking and oral contraceptives.
   b. Drug therapy
      Indications for drug therapy include family history of early complications of hypertension, target organ damage (e.g., ocular, cardiac, renal, CNS), and symptoms or signs related to elevated BP. The stepped-care approach is popular.

TABLE 7-14.

Routine and Special Laboratory Tests and Their Significance

Laboratory Test	Significance of Abnormal Results
Urinalysis, urine culture, BUN, creatinine, uric acid	Renal parenchymal disease
Serum electrolytes (hypokalemia)	Hyperaldosteronism, primary or secondary Adrenogenital syndrome Renin-producing tumors
ECG, CXR film, echo	Cardiac cause of hypertension, also baseline function
IV pyelography (or ultrasonography, radionuclide studies, CT of kidneys)	Renal parenchymal disease Renovascular hypertension Tumors (neuroblastoma, Wilms tumor)
Plasma renin activity (PRA), peripheral	High-renin hypertension Renovascular hypertension Renin-producing tumors Some Cushing syndrome Some essential hypertension Low-renin hypertension Adrenogenital syndrome Primary hyperaldosteronism
24-hr urine collection for 17-KS and 17-OHCS	Cushing syndrome Adrenogenital syndrome
24-hr urine collection for catecholamines and VMA	Pheochromocytoma Neuroblastoma
Aldosterone	Hyperaldosteronism, primary or secondary Renovascular hypertension Renin-producing tumors
Renal vein PRA	Unilateral renal parenchymal disease Renovascular hypertension
Abdominal aortogram	Renovascular hypertension Abdominal coarctation of aorta Unilateral renal parenchymal diseases Pheochromocytoma

Step 1: A small dose of a single antihypertensive drug, either a diuretic (e.g., hydrochlorothiazide, chlorothiazide, furosemide, spironolactone) or an adrenergic inhibitor (e.g., propranolol, atenolol, metoprolol, methyldopa, prazosine) is followed by a full dose, if necessary. In a black, diabetic, or asthmatic patient, the diuretic is suggested as first-step therapy. A β-adrenergic blocker may be contraindicated in diabetics and asthmatics; the diuretic works well in adult black patients. In adolescents with hyperdynamic-type hypertension (with a rapid pulse) or one associated with hyperthyroidism, a β-blocker is preferable.

Step 2: If the first drug is not effective, a second drug may be added to or substituted for the first drug, starting with a small dose and proceeding to a full dose.

Step 3: If BP still remains high, a third drug, usually a vasodilator (hydralazine, minoxidil, or captopril), may be added to the regimen. Dosages of commonly used antihypertensive drugs for children appear in Table 7-15.

Recently, calcium antagonists are being used increasingly in the treatment of adult hypertension, but there is limited experience with children. Nifedipine has the greatest peripheral vasodilatory action and little effect on cardiac automaticity, conduction, or contractility. Concomitant dietary sodium restriction or the use of a diuretic agent may not be necessary, as calcium antagonists cause natriuresis by producing renal vasodilation. The starting adult dose is 10 mg three times a day, which may be titrated up to 20 to 30 mg three times a day.

2. Secondary hypertension: Treatment of secondary hypertension should be aimed at removing the cause whenever possible. The medical management discussed in the previous section can control hypertension caused by most renal parenchymal diseases. Concomitant antibiotic therapy for infectious processes may be indicated. Unilateral renal parenchymal dis-

TABLE 7-15.

Recommended Oral Dosages of Selected Antihypertensive Drugs for Children

Drugs	Dose (mg/kg)	Times/day
Diuretics		
Hydrochlorothiazide (HydroDiuril)	1-2	2
Chlorothiazide (Diuril)	0.5-2	1
Furosemide (Lasix)	0.5-2	2
Spironolactone (Aldactone)	1-2	2
Adrenergic Inhibitors		
Propranolol (Inderal)	1-3	3
Methyldopa (Aldomet)	5-10	2
Atenolol (Tenormin)	1-2	1
Vasodilators		
Hydralazine (Apresoline)	1-5	2-3
Minoxidil (Loniten)	0.1-1	2
ACE Inhibitors		
Captopril (Capoten)		
<6 mo	0.05-0.5	3
>6 mo	0.5-2.0	3

Modified from the Second NIH Task Force on Blood Pressure Control in Children, Pediatrics 79:1, 1987.

ease may be treated with a unilateral nephrectomy. Renovascular disease may be cured by successful surgery (e.g., reconstruction of a stenotic renal artery, autotransplantation, or unilateral nephrectomy). Hypertension caused by tumors (pheochromocytoma, neuroblastoma) are treated primarily by surgery. Surgical repair or balloon angioplasty is indicated for COA.

Hypertensive Crisis

1. In a patient with severe hypertension (above 180 mm Hg systolic or 110 mm Hg diastolic), any of the following features indicates a hypertensive emergency:
   a. Neurologic signs with severe headache, vomiting, irritability or apathy, seizures, papilledema, retinal

       hemorrhage, or exudate (hypertensive encepha-
       lopathy).
  b. CHF or pulmonary edema.
2. Aggressive parenteral administration of antihyperten-
    sive drugs is indicated to lower blood pressure.
    a. Diazoxide (Hyperstat) 1 to 3 mg/kg as an IV bolus
       or nitroprusside (Nipride) 2 to 3 mg/kg/min as an
       IV drip.
    b. If hypertension is less severe, hydralazine (Apreso-
       line) 0.15 mg/kg IV or IM may be used. The dose
       may be repeated at 4 to 6 hour intervals.
    c. A rapid-acting diuretic such as furosemide 1 mg/
       kg is given IV to initiate diuresis.
    d. Fluid balance must be controlled carefully so that
       intake is limited to urine output plus insensible
       loss.
    e. Seizures may be treated with slow IV infusion of di-
       azepam (Valium) 0.2 mg/kg or other anticonvul-
       sant medication.
    f. When a hypertensive crisis is under control, oral
       medications will replace the parenteral medica-
       tions (see Chapter 9, Cardiovascular Drug Dosage).

VI. HYPERLIPIDEMIA IN CHILDHOOD

It is widely believed that atherosclerotic lesions start to develop
in childhood and progress to irreversible lesions in adulthood. High levels of total cholesterol, low-density lipoprotein
(LDL), and very low density lipoprotein (VLDL) and low
levels of high-density lipoprotein (HDL) are correlated with
an increased risk for coronary heart disease in adolescents and
young adults. Since substantial and potentially irreversible
atherosclerosis may already exist by the fourth decade of life,
efforts to lower serum cholesterol levels in children have been
made in the hope of preventing or retarding the progress of
atherosclerosis. Recently the National Cholesterol Education
Program Expert Panel on Blood Cholesterol Levels in Children and Adolescents (1991, NIH Publication No. 91-2732)
has recommended strategies for prevention and detection of
hyperlipidemia in children (see later section).

TABLE 7-16.

Other Risk Factors for Early Onset of Coronary Heart Disease

---

1. Family history of premature coronary heart disease, cerebro-vascular or occlusive peripheral vascular disease (with onset before age 55 for men and before age 65 for women in a sibling, parent, or sibling of a parent).
2. Cigarette smoking.
3. Hypertension.
4. Low HDL cholesterol (<35 mg/dl).
5. Diabetes mellitus.
6. Physical inactivity.

Adapted from Summary of the Second Report of the National Cholesterol Education Program (NCEP) Expert Panel on Detection, Evaluation, and Treatment of High Blood Cholesterol in Adults (Adult Treatment Panel II), JAMA 269:3015-3023, 1993.

Reduction of elevated cholesterol is only one aspect of the total management plan. Other interrelated factors such as genetics, hypertension, diabetes mellitus, obesity, and smoking are important risk factors in the development of athero-sclerotic cardiovascular disease (Table 7-16). Physicians should play an increasing role not only in the detection of hyperlipidemia, but also in counseling for prevention of other risk factors.

A. Clinical Features of Hypercholesterolemia

1. Secondary hypercholesterolemia: All children with LDL cholesterol levels of 130 mg/dl or more should be evaluated for possible secondary hypercholesterol-emia (Table 7-17). The usual causes of secondary hypercholesterolemia in children are obesity and the use of oral contraceptives, isotretinoin (Accutane), or anabolic steroids. In addition to a careful history and physical examination, determination of blood glucose and appropriate tests of liver, kidney, and thyroid function may be indicated.
2. Primary hypercholesterolemia: If secondary causes of hypercholesterolemia are excluded, primary hy-

TABLE 7-17.

Causes of Secondary Hypercholesterolemia

Exogenous Causes
Drugs: corticosteroids, isotretinoin (Accutane), thiazides, anticonvulsants, β-blockers, anabolic steroids, certain oral contraceptives
Alcohol
Obesity

Endocrine and Metabolic Disorders
Hypothyroidism
Diabetes mellitus
Lipodystrophy
Pregnancy
Idiopathic hypercalcemia
Glycogen storage diseases
Sphingolipidoses

Obstructive Liver Diseases
Biliary atresia
Biliary cirrhosis

Chronic Renal Diseases
Nephrotic syndrome

Miscellaneous Causes
Anorexia nervosa
Progeria
Collagen diseases
Klinefelter syndrome

percholesterolemia is considered present. Screening of all family members is recommended to determine whether the disorder is familial. Family screening is important not only for detection of hypercholesterolemia in other members of the family but also in emphasizing the need for the entire family to change their eating patterns. Young patients found to have elevated LDL cholesterol are more likely to have a familial disorder of LDL metabolism. The two most common familial lipoprotein disorders with elevated LDL cholesterol are familial hypercholesterolemia (FH) and familial combined hyperlipidemia (FCH).

Familial Hypercholesterolemia

FH, a disorder of lipoprotein metabolism, is due to absence or reduction of LDL receptors. Heterozygotes have about 50% reduction in LDL receptors, and homozygotes have little or no receptor activity. This autosomal-dominant condition is fairly common, occurring in 1 in 500 people. An evaluation of the family members is important to the diagnosis. One of the parents and one of two siblings will have elevated total and LDL cholesterol levels, while the unaffected first-degree relatives will have completely normal levels.

Heterozygotes have total and LDL cholesterol levels two to three times normal. Their total cholesterol levels are most often above 240 mg/dl (average 300 mg/dl), and their LDL cholesterol levels are above 160 mg/dl (average 240 mg/dl). The triglyceride levels are usually normal. Extensor tendon xanthomas in the parents of such children almost confirm the diagnosis. A heterozygote child or adolescent will have normal physical findings; tendon xanthomas are rarely found in anyone under age 10, and only about 10% to 15% develop them in the second decade, primarily in the Achilles tendons and extensor tendons of the hands.

Homozygote children, who have inherited two mutant FH genes, occur rarely (one in a million). Their total and LDL cholesterol levels are five to six time normal. Such children have cholesterol levels that average about 700 mg/dl but may reach 1 g/dl or higher. Clinical signs such as planar xanthomas and flat orange-colored skin lesions in the webbing of the hands and over the elbows and buttocks may be present by the time the patient reaches age 5. Tendon xanthomas, corneal arcus, and clinically significant coronary heart disease are often present by the time the patient is age 10. The generalized atherosclerosis often affects the aortic valve, causing aortic stenosis.

Familial Combined Hyperlipidemia

Familial combined hyperlipidemia (FCH) is more common than FH, possibly occurring in 1 in 300 people. Clinically it may be difficult to separate this entity from FH. Most patients with FCH lack tendon xanthomas, and extreme hyperlipidemia is absent in childhood. FCH is suggested by (1) elevated triglyceride levels in parents with hypercholesterolemia, (2) moderately elevated triglyceride levels (average 120 mg/dl for boys and 130 mg/dl for girls), (3) somewhat lower levels of total and LDL cholesterol than in those with FH, and (4) LDL levels that fluctuate, with triglyceride levels fluctuating in the opposite direction. Such children usually have a plasma total cholesterol level between 190 and 220 mg/dl. The LDL cholesterol level is usually normal or only mildly elevated.

B. Cholesterol-Lowering Strategies

The Expert Panel (NIH Publication No 91-2732, September 1991) has recommended two complementary approaches, population and individualized, to lower blood cholesterol levels for children and adolescents. The following are excerpts from the recommendations.

1. The population approach: For children older than age 2, the following are recommended:
   a. Nutritional adequacy should be achieved by eating a wide variety of foods.
   b. Adequate calories should be provided for normal growth and development.
   c. The following pattern of nutrient intake is recommended (Step One diet, Table 7-18): saturated fatty acids less than 10% of total calories, total fat not more than 30% of total calories, and dietary cholesterol less than 300 mg per day. Children younger than age 2 may require a higher percentage of calories from fat.
2. The individualized approach: This is to identify and treat children and adolescents who are at high risk for having high cholesterol levels.
   Selective Screening: The Expert Panel recommends selective screening of children and adolescents with a family history of premature cardiovascular disease (or at least one parent with high serum cholesterol).
   1) Children and adolescents whose parents or grandparents at age 55 or less (for men)

TABLE 7-18.

Nutrient Composition of Step One and Step Two Diets

Nutrient	Step One Diet	Step Two Diet
Total fat (% total calories)	<30%	<30%
Saturated fatty acids	<10%	<7%
Polyunsaturated fatty acids	≤10%	≤10%
Monounsaturated fatty acids	10%-15%	10%-15%
Carbohydrates (% of total calories)	50%-60%	50%-60%
Protein (% of total calories)	10%-20%	10%-20%
Cholesterol (per day)	<300 mg	<200 mg
Total calories	To achieve and maintain desirable weight	To achieve and maintain desirable weight

and 65 years or less (for women*) were found to have coronary atherosclerosis following angiography or underwent balloon angioplasty or coronary artery bypass surgery.

2) Children and adolescents whose parents or grandparents at age 55 years or less (for men) and age 65 years or less (for women*) had documented myocardial infarction, angina pectoris, peripheral vascular disease, cerebrovascular disease, or sudden cardiac death.

3) The offspring of a parent who has been found to have high total cholesterol (240 mg/dl or higher).

4) Children and adolescents whose parental or grandparental history is unobtainable, particularly patients with other risk factors.

The recommendations of selective screening are somewhat controversial.

*The new guidelines by the Expert Panel of National Cholesterol Education Program (June 1993).

Several recent studies support universal screening. Optional cholesterol testing by the practicing physician may be appropriate for certain children who are judged to be at high risk for coronary heart disease (for such reasons as smoking, high blood pressure, obesity, or excessive amount of fat intake).

Total Cholesterol Level or Lipoprotein Profile: The panel's recommendations vary according to the reasons for testing.

1) For young people being tested because they have at least one parent with a high blood cholesterol, the initial step is a measurement of total cholesterol.

2) For children who have a family history of premature cardiovascular disease, a lipoprotein analysis is recommended, because a high proportion of these children have some lipoprotein abnormalities.

Classification: Depending on the total cholesterol and LDL cholesterol levels, patients are categorized as *acceptable, borderline,* or *high.*

1) For those who had total cholesterol levels mcasured, acceptable is less than 170 mg/dl; borderline is 170 to 199 mg/dl; and high is above 200 mg/dl. Recommendations for each category are given in Fig 7-1.

2) For those who had lipoprotein analysis done: Regardless of indications, a lipoprotein analysis should be repeated and the average LDL cholesterol levels determined. The patient is then categorized as acceptable (LDL cholesterol below 110 mg/dl), borderline (110 to 129 mg/dl), and high (130 mg/dl or higher). Recommendations for each category are given in Fig 7-2.

3. Measurements of cholesterol and lipoproteins

a. Total cholesterol and LDL cholesterol levels are not measured before the person is age 2, and no treatment is recommended before that age. Levels are reasonably consistent thereafter (with some small increment during adolescence).

Text continued on p. 286.

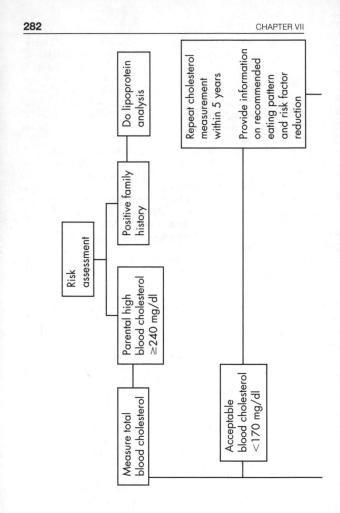

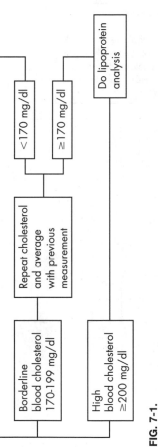

FIG. 7-1.
Risk assessment recommended by the Expert Panel on Blood Cholesterol Levels in Children and Adolescents, National Cholesterol Education Program (NIH Publication No 91-2732, September, 1991).

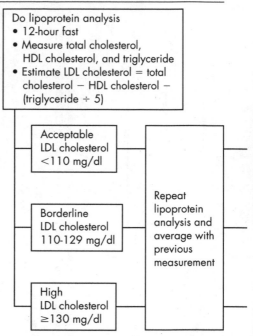

FIG. 7-2.
Classification, education, and follow-up based on LDL cholesterol, recommended by the Expert Panel on Blood Cholesterol Levels in Children and Adolescents, National Cholesterol Education Program (NIH Publication No 91-2732, September, 1991).

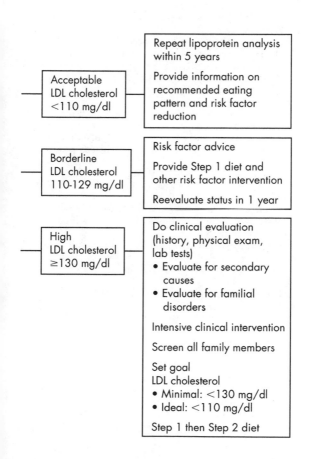

Acceptable
LDL cholesterol
<110 mg/dl

Repeat lipoprotein analysis
within 5 years

Provide information on
recommended eating
pattern and risk factor
reduction

Borderline
LDL cholesterol
110-129 mg/dl

Risk factor advice

Provide Step 1 diet and
other risk factor intervention

Reevaluate status in 1 year

High
LDL cholesterol
≥130 mg/dl

Do clinical evaluation
(history, physical exam,
lab tests)
• Evaluate for secondary
  causes
• Evaluate for familial
  disorders

Intensive clinical intervention

Screen all family members

Set goal
LDL cholesterol
• Minimal: <130 mg/dl
• Ideal: <110 mg/dl

Step 1 then Step 2 diet

   b. The child does not have to be fasting for measurement of total cholesterol.

   c. A lipoprotein analysis is obtained after an overnight fast of 12 hours. Total cholesterol, HDL cholesterol and triglyceride levels are measured. The LDL cholesterol level is then estimated by the Friedewald formula:

      LDL cholesterol = total cholesterol − HDL cholesterol − (triglyceride ÷ 5). This formula is not accurate if the child is not fasting, if the triglyceride level is above 400 mg/dl, or if chylomicrons or dysbetalipoproteinemia is present.

Treatment

  Diet Therapy: Diet therapy is prescribed in two steps that progressively reduce the intake of saturated fatty acids and cholesterol. Involvement of a registered dietitian or other qualified health professional is recommended.

1. The Step One Diet (Table 7-18) contains the same nutrient intake recommended in the population approach to lowering cholesterol.

2. If the Step One Diet for 3 months fails to achieve the minimal goals of therapy, the Step Two Diet is prescribed (Table 7-18).

  Drug Therapy: The Expert Panel recommends drug therapy in children ages 10 years and older if after an adequate trial of diet therapy (6 months to 1 year):

   a. LDL cholesterol remains 190 mg/dl or higher, or

   b. LDL cholesterol remains 160 mg/dl or higher *and*

     1) There is a family history of premature cardiovascular disease (before age 55 in men and before age 65 in women), *or*

     2) Two or more other cardiovascular disease risk factors (such as HDL cholesterol below 35 mg/dl, cigarette smoking, high blood pressure, obesity or diabetes) are present.

    For children and adolescents with hypercholesterolemia, only the bile acid sequestrants (cholestyramine, colestipol) are recommended. The bile acid sequestrants increase excretion of bile acids in stool and increase LDL receptor activity. Niacin, HMG CoA (3-hydroxy-3 methylglutaryl-coenzyme A) reductase inhibitors (lovastatin, pravastatin), probucol, fibric acid derivatives (gemfibrozil, clofibrate) are not recommended as routine drugs for use in children and adolescents.

MANAGEMENT OF CARDIAC SURGICAL PATIENTS

VIII

The current trend is to carry out total repair of CHDs at an early age whenever such repair is technically possible. Early total repair obviates the need for palliative procedures and possibly prevents permanent damage to the cardiovascular system, which is known to develop in certain CHDs. However, recommendations for the timing and type of operation vary from institution to institution. The improved results currently seen with pediatric cardiac surgery are in part attributed to improved surgical technique and perioperative care.

Open heart procedures use cardiopulmonary bypass (CPB) with some degree of hypothermia and a varying duration of circulatory arrest. Open procedures are required for repair of intracardiac anomalies (e.g., VSD, TOF, TGA). Closed procedures do not require CPB; they are performed for repair of extracardiac anomalies (e.g., COA, PDA) or palliative procedures (e.g., S-P shunt procedures or PA banding). The following sections outline some pertinent aspects of preoperative and postoperative management of cardiac patients for pediatricians.

I. PREOPERATIVE MANAGEMENT

Good preoperative preparation is important for a smooth operative and postoperative course.

1. All children should have a careful history and physical examination 1 or 2 days before surgery. This is to gain

a full understanding of chronic medical problems and to uncover acute medical problems (e.g., pneumonia, upper respiratory infections, otitis media) that would mandate cancellation of elective surgery.

2. Laboratory evaluation
   a. Complete blood count, urinalysis, serum electrolytes, serum glucose, and blood urea nitrogen (BUN) of all cardiac patients are routinely obtained.
   b. CXR film and ECG of all patients are obtained.
   c. For open heart procedures, blood coagulation studies—prothrombin time (PT), partial thromboplastin time (PTT), and platelet count—are obtained.

3. All patients undergoing CPB are cross-matched for six units of blood. One to two units of blood are cross-matched for those undergoing closed procedures.

4. Medications
   a. Digoxin is discontinued after the evening dose.
   b. Diuretics are discontinued 8 to 12 hours preoperatively (or this may be individualized).
   c. Propranolol and antiarrhythmics are continued at the same dosage until immediately before the surgery.
   d. Nonsteroidal antiinflammatory drugs (aspirin, indomethacin, ibuprofen) and antiplatelet drugs (persantin) are discontinued 7 or more days prior to surgery.

5. Prevention of infection
   Broad-spectrum antibiotics are used to decrease the risk of perioperative infection. These are continued through postoperative day 3 or until 24 hours after removal of all chest tubes and intracardiac and vascular monitoring lines.
   a. Cefazolin (Ancef or Kefzol) (or equivalent cephalosporin) 75 to 100 mg/kg/day (maximum 6 g/24 hr) IV q8h starting immediately prior to surgery is a popular regimen.
   b. Vancomycin 10 to 15 mg/kg/dose IV q8h is used for patients with known penicillin allergy.

   c. For newborns, gentamicin 2.5 mg/kg/dose IV q8h along with nafcillin 50 mg/kg/day IV q8h may be used.

6. For older children, the emotional preparation for surgery is as important as the physical preparation.

II. POSTOPERATIVE CARE OF CARDIAC PATIENTS

A high level of vigilance for signs of complications should be maintained during the postoperative period so that appropriate therapy can be initiated early.

A. Normal Convalescence

Physicians should be familiar with the postoperative course of normally convalescing patients in order to recognize abnormal convalescence.

1. Cardiovascular system
   a. Warm skin, full peripheral pulses with brisk capillary refill, normal BP and an adequate urine output (at least 1 ml/kg/hr) are clinical evidence of good cardiac output. Measured cardiac index by thermodilution method should be greater than 2 L/min/m^2.
   b. Mild arterial hypertension is present in early postoperative period following CPB (because of increased levels of catecholamines, plasma renin, or angiotensin II).
   c. Cardiac rhythm should be sinus and the heart rate relatively high. Ranges of heart rate (beats/min) in normally convalescing postoperative patients are as follows:

less than 6 months	110 to 190
6 to 12 months	100 to 170
1 to 3 years	90 to 160
over 3 years	80 to 150

2. Pulmonary system
   a. Arterial blood gases are in the acceptable normal range.

    b. CXR films show no evidence of pneumothorax, atelectasis, or pleural effusion.

3. Renal system: Adequate urine output (i.e., above 1 ml/kg/hr) and evidence of adequate solute excretion (e.g., serum K below 5 mEq/L; BUN below 40 mg/dl; creatinine below 1 mg/dl) are signs of normal renal function.

4. Metabolic system
    a. Retention of water and sodium and depletion of whole body potassium are commonly seen following open heart surgery. They result in mild hyponatremia and hypokalemia and 5% weight gain.
    b. Mild metabolic acidosis (with base deficit of −4 mEq/L) is common in the first few hours after CPB and does not require treatment.
    c. Varying degrees of fever (up to 39.5°C or 103°F) are nearly always present during the first 4 or 5 days, and extensive work-up for infection is not indicated. Causes of fever include reaction to CPB, infection, reaction to homologous blood, atelectasis, pleural effusion, low cardiac output, and brain stem damage.

5. Hematologic system: clotting studies should be normal and hemoglobin should be at least 9.5 g/dl or higher.

6. Neurologic: The patient should respond appropriately for the level of sedation without evidence of neurologic defects (e.g., hemiplegia, visual field defects) or seizures.

B. Care Following Uncomplicated Operation

1. General care
    a. Fluid replacement: Because of the tendency to retain sodium and water, a minimal amount of dextrose in water (D_5W in infants, $D_{10}W$ in children), without sodium is administered for approximately 48 hours after surgery. A modest amount of potassium (10 mEq/m^2/day) is given on the first day of surgery. Recommended fluid volume replace-

ments in the first 24 hours after open procedures are as follows:

60 ml/kg for first 10 kg of body weight (BW)

30 ml/kg for second 10 kg of BW

15 ml/kg for remainder of BW

After closed procedures 160% of these amounts may be given.

b. The patient should receive medications for sedation and adequate pain relief. Morphine sulfate IV drip at 0.025 to 2 mg/kg/hr (or 0.1 to 0.2 mg/kg/dose q3h) or fentanyl at 2 to 10 µg/kg/hr (or 1 to 2 µg/kg/dose q30-60min) are commonly used.

c. Measures to prevent pulmonary hypertensive crisis are important for patients who had severe pulmonary hypertension preoperatively. The following are recommended:

1) Paralysis by pancuronium bromide (continuous IV drip at 0.1 mg/kg/hr or intermittent IV infusion of 0.1 mg/kg/dose q30-60min).

2) Intravenous nitroprusside or nitroglycerin and inhaled nitric oxide.

3) A longer duration of intubation until the cardiac and respiratory functions are stable.

2. Pulmonary system

a. Extubated patients should show no signs of respiratory distress (grunting, nasal flaring, and retraction). Good chest expansion and evidence of good air exchange to both lungs should be present. All patients are placed in an oxygen mist environment at a fractional inspired oxygen concentration (Fio_2) of 0.5. Pulmonary physiotherapy (consisting of coughing and deep breathing exercise and positional changes with or without clapping and vibrating) is administered every 4 hours.

b. In intubated patients, CXR films are obtained to check the position of chest tubes and central and arterial lines and to check for evidence of pneumothorax, atelectasis, pleural effusion, or main stem bronchus intubation. Significant degrees of pneumothorax or pleural effusion may require treatment. Widening of the mediastinal shadow suggests accumulation of blood and requires investigation of the function of the mediastinal chest tube.

The respiratory rate (15 to 30 breaths/min), Fio_2 (0.5 to 1) and tidal volume (10 to 15 ml/kg) are set to maintain the partial pressure of oxygen (Po_2) at 70 to 100 mm Hg, the pH at 7.35 to 7.45, and the partial pressure of carbon dioxide (Pco_2) at 30 to 40 mm Hg. In the first postoperative days the goal of ventilation is to maintain adequate oxygenation (Po_2 100 to 150 mm Hg) and mild respiratory alkalosis (pH 7.5 to 7.65) along with a Pco_2 between 28 and 35 mm Hg (all to decrease PVR). Hyperventilation (Pco_2 below 30 mm Hg) is corrected by decreasing the ventilator rate, decreasing the tidal volume and adding dead space (5 to 10 ml at a time) to the airway. Hypoventilation is corrected by the opposite maneuvers. Low Po_2 is corrected by raising the Fio_2, adding positive end-expiratory pressure (PEEP), or increasing tidal volume. Physiologic PEEP of 3 to 5 cm H_2O is used in children. The use of a high mean airway pressure or high levels of PEEP may increase PVR and decrease cardiac output; both should be avoided in a patient who has had a Senning, Fontan, or Glenn operation.

Tracheal toilet is carried out through the endotracheal tube every 2 hours, or more often if necessary. It consists of instillation of 0.5 to 5 ml of saline and suctioning of both main-stem bronchi and ventilation by Ambu bag for 1 to 2 minutes with oxygen (Fio_2 1) immediately before and after suctioning.

c. Extubation is performed as soon as possible, usually in the operating room in children undergoing closed procedures, within 4 to 8 hours after uncomplicated open heart procedures, and the day after complex open procedures. Criteria for extubation include the following:

1) The patient should be awake and alert.

2) The patient should be breathing well, with a spontaneous respiratory rate of 40 breaths/min in young children and 50 breaths/min in infants, without the use of accessory respiratory muscles. Under a minimal ventilator setting (with Fio_2 no more than 0.4, tidal volume at 8 to 10 ml/kg, and PEEP no more than 5 cm H_2O) there should be no evidence of hypoxia or hypercarbia.

3) The patient should be in a satisfactory and stable hemodynamic state (normal BP, adequate cardiac output, no significant arrhythmias).

4) The patient should not have important bleeding (and should have minimal chest tube drainage).

Postextubation subglottitis is treated with racemic epinephrine nebulizer (0.125 to 0.5 ml of 2.25% recemic epinephrine, diluted with 2 to 3 ml of water or normal saline administered by aerosol).

3. Cardiovascular system: Complete correction of the intracardiac defect and adequate intraoperative myocardial protection generally will result in good cardiac function after surgery. Signs of reduced cardiac output, abnormal blood pressures or heart rate, and abnormal rhythm should be continually monitored.

a. Inadequate cardiac output is the most frequent and serious sign of abnormal convalescence. The following are signs of low cardiac output: (1) cold extremities and weak pulses, (2) oliguria (urine output below 1 ml/kg/hr), (3) rising serum K levels (to 5 mEq/L), (4) partial venous pressure of oxygen (Pvo_2) from RA or central venous line below 28 mm Hg, and/or (5) measured cardiac index below 2 $L/min/m^2$.

Inadequate cardiac output may be caused by (1) low preload (low atrial or central venous pressure), (2) high afterload, (3) depressed myocardial contractility, (4) cardiac tamponade (5) brachycardia or extreme tachycardia, and (6) inadequate surgical repair. Treatment is directed at the cause.

1) In general, atrial pressures are directly related to intravascular blood volume and inversely re-

lated to ventricular compliance. Low preload (or low atrial pressure) is treated with an increase in blood volume to raise either the right or left atrial pressure to 15 to 20 mm Hg in children (and 10 to 15 mm Hg in infants). RA pressure may be raised to 25 to 30 mm Hg in children after TOF repair.

2) High afterload (with increased SVR) may be caused by hypoxia, acidosis, hypothermia, or pain. In addition to the correction of the cause, the elevated SVR may be treated with vasodilators (nitroprusside or nitroglycerin) or morphine infusion. Nitroprusside (Nipride) has a favorable effect on the PVR; nitroglycerin is also a potent coronary vasodilator.

3) Depressed myocardial contractility (demonstrated by echo) may be treated by improving arterial oxygen saturation or inotropic agents. The former is achieved by maintaining a patent airway with good respiratory care, increasing Fio_2 if necessary, reducing pulmonary shunting by the use of PEEP, and reducing pulmonary edema by the use of diuretics. The following inotropic agents may be used:

   a) Dopamine starting at 2.5 µg/kg/min and increasing up to 15 µg/kg/min if necessary.

   b) Epinephrine, isoproterenol, or dobutamine may be gradually added if dopamine is not effective.

   c) Amrinone, a noncatecholamine inotropic agent with vasodilator effects, may be used alone or added to the regimen.

4) Cardiac tamponade is treated with an urgent decompression of the pericardial space. Early cardiac tamponade results from persistent surgical bleeding not properly drained by the chest tubes: it may even occur when the pericardium is removed or left widely open. It must be suspected when the chest tube drainage abruptly decreases or stops in a patient with previous significant

bleeding. Characteristically the arterial pressure falls and shows a minimal response to volume administration. Cardiac tamponade requires prompt surgical exploration for evacuation of the pericardial hematoma or control of bleeding by an urgent opening of the sternotomy, often in the intensive care unit. When time permits, echo may demonstrate cardiac tamponade.

5) Bradycardia is treated with atrial or ventricular pacing or chronotropic agents. Atrial and ventricular pacing wires are routinely placed at the time of open heart procedures and are left for 5 to 7 days postoperatively. Extreme tachycardia is treated by eliminating causes if known (fever, volume depletion, or arrhythmias).

6) Immediate surgical repair is occasionally indicated when an inadequate surgical repair (such as a large residual L-R shunt or an R-L shunt) is the cause of low cardiac output.

7) *Pulmonary hypertensive crisis* is characterized by an acute rise in PA pressure followed by a reduction in cardiac output and a fall in arterial oxygen saturation. It occurs in neonates and infants who had CHDs with pulmonary hypertension (e.g., complete ECD, persistent truncus arteriosus), often after suctioning of the endotracheal tube. It is difficult to treat and may be fatal; prevention is critically important (see General Care earlier in this chapter). Treatment includes hyperventilation with 100% oxygen, sedation with IV fentanyl or morphine, and paralysis with IV pancuronium.

b. Hypotension and hypertension

1) Hypotension with blood pressures at the lower ranges of normal is treated with a volume expander, initially 10 to 20 ml/kg. If that fails to raise BP, inotropic agents are used. $CaCl_2$ may be helpful in treating hypotension (since citrated blood given to the patient binds ionized calcium).

2) Severe hypertension is treated with vasodilators.

    c. Rhythm disorders: Sinus rhythm is optimal. Nodal (or AV junctional) rhythm may reduce cardiac output by 10% to 15%. In addition to the specific treatment for arrhythmias, possible causes should be investigated and corrected, e.g., via evaluation of oxygenation, ventilator function, acid-base status, serum K, and the dosages of cardiotonic agents.

      1) Frequent PVCs (more than 6/min) are treated with lidocaine 1 mg/kg IV. PVCs associated with hypokalemia may be eliminated by IV supplementary potassium.

      2) Ventricular tachycardia is treated with lidocaine, DC cardioversion, or overdrive suppression.

      3) Atrial fibrillation is treated with digoxin (in stable patients) or cardioversion (in hemodynamically compromised patients).

      4) Atrial flutter is treated with overdrive suppression or cardioversion and digoxin (for 8 weeks) to prevent recurrences.

      5) SVT is treated with adenosine (the drug of choice). It may also be treated with overdrive suppression or cardioversion. Propranolol or verapamil IV may be used with caution. Digoxin is given for 8 weeks to prevent recurrences.

      6) AV dissociation is treated with sequential atrioventricular pacing using temporary epicardial pacing wires placed at the time of surgery.

      7) Complete heart block is treated by temporary pacing and/or isoproterenol. A permanent pacemaker should be inserted if normal sinus rhythm has not returned within 14 days of surgery.

4. Renal system

Oliguria (below 1 ml/kg/hr) and evidence of solute accumulation (serum K above 5 mEq/L, BUN above 40 mg/dl, creatinine above 1 mg/dl) indicate acute renal failure. Acute reduction of cardiac output is the most common cause of renal failure. Initial treatment is directed at improving cardiac output and inducing diuresis.

    a. Preload and afterload should be optimized and do-
       pamine infusion used.

    b. Furosemide (Lasix) 1 mg/kg q4-6h IV. If no re-
       sponse, 2 mg/kg and then 4 mg/kg may be used
       for 3 days.

    c. If serum K rises above 6.5 mEq/L, glucose-insulin
       solution (0.5 g glucose/kg with 0.3 U crystalline
       insulin/g of glucose, given IV over 2 hours) and
       sodium polystyrene sulfonate (Kayexalate) enema
       are used.

    d. Peritoneal dialysis may be necessary if those mea-
       sures are ineffective. Indications for peritoneal di-
       alysis include BUN over 100 mg/dl, life-threaten-
       ing hyperkalemia, intractable metabolic acidosis,
       pulmonary compromise, or fluid restrictions limit-
       ing caloric intake.

5. Metabolic system

    a. Abnormalities of electrolytes and acid-base balance

       1) Mild hyponatremia does not require treatment
          except for fluid restriction and diuretics. Serum
          Na below 125 mEq/L requires treatment to el-
          evate sodium levels.

       2) Hypernatremia with the serum Na above 155
          mEq/L requires treatment with sodium restric-
          tion and liberalization of fluids.

       3) Metabolic acidosis is treated if the base deficit
          is above –5 mEq/L.

Total extracellular base deficit = base deficit
      (mEq/L) × 0.3 × BW (kg).

       The dosage of sodium bicarbonate is half of the
       total extracellular base deficit.

    b. Treat hypoglycemia (below 50 mg/dl) or hypocal-
       cemia (total calcium below 8 mg/dl, ionized cal-
       cium below 4 mg/dl).

    c. Fever above 38.5°C (101.3°F) is treated as follows:

       1) Acetaminophen suppository 10 mg/kg q4h.

       2) Dexamethasone 0.25 mg/kg IV and then 0.1
          mg/kg IV q6h × 4 (for possible transfusion re-
          action).

      3) Cooling blanket if the temperature is above 39.8°C (103.6°F) and not responding to acetaminophen.

      4) Sodium nitroprusside to increase peripheral heat loss.

      5) Pancuronium to reduce muscle heat production.

  d. Nutrition: Oral feeding is begun in infants 8 hours after extubation, starting with glucose water q4h and advancing to an appropriate formula. Gavage feeding should be used if the baby is too weak to suck. Infants with prolonged intubation require gavage feeding or total parenteral nutrition.

6. Hematologic system

  a. Maintain adequate hemoglobin (Hgb) and a desirable filling pressure (e.g., LA pressure 6 to 14 mm Hg) by infusion of packed cells, salt-poor albumin, or plasma, depending on the patient's Hgb or hematocrit (Hct). Packed cells are given when Hgb is below 10 g/dl (or Hct below 30%); colloid solutions are given when Hgb is over 10 g/dl (or Hct over 30%).

  b. Coagulation abnormalities may result from inadequate heparin neutralization (causing prolongation of PTT), thrombocytopenia (below 50,000 platelets/mm^3) or disseminated intravascular coagulation (DIC, usually associated with bacteremia and prolonged low cardiac output state). Unneutralized heparin is corrected by administration of additional protamine. Thrombocytopenia is treated with slow infusion of platelet concentrates with an infusion pump, given over 20 to 30 min; rapid infusion may cause pulmonary hypertension and RV failure.

  c. Excessive postoperative bleeding occurs more frequently in severely cyanotic patients, polycythemic patients, and patients who had a reoperation. Necessity to infuse more than 10 to 15 ml/kg of volume requires investigation for excessive blood loss and for a possible surgical reexploration.

Surgical reexploration is indicated (1) if the chest tube drainage in the absence of clotting abnormalities exceeds 3 ml/kg/hr for 3 hours or (2) if there is a sudden marked increase in chest tube drainage of 5 ml/kg/hr in any 1 hour.

7. Gastrointestinal system: Evidence of abdominal distention, absence of peristalsis, and hyperperistalsis is sought twice a day. If one of these develops, alimentation is discontinued and IV hyperalimentation is considered. Gastrointestinal (GI) dysfunction may be caused by GI bleeding, acute pancreatitis, hepatic necrosis, intestinal necrosis, constipation, ileus, and others. Cimetidine may be administered prophylactically to patients with or without a history of peptic ulcer disease.

8. Neurologic system
   a. Localized neurologic defects such as hemiplegia and visual field defects are abnormal and may be due to air or particulate emboli.
   b. Seizures may be caused by metabolic abnormalities, infections, cerebral edema, embolism or hemorrhage, or decreased cerebral perfusion. Seizures seldom have ominous long-term complications. Management of seizures includes the following:
      1) Determine arterial blood gases, serum glucose, calcium and electrolytes, cardiac output, and temperature. Correct any abnormalities.
      2) Anticonvulsant therapy
         a) Valium 0.1 to 0.2 mg/kg IV if the patient is being ventilated (valium has respiratory depressant effects).
         b) Phenobarbital 10 to 15 mg/kg IV over 5 to 10 min. (The full effect may take several hours.)
         c) Dilantin 20 mg/kg PO followed by a maintenance dose of 3 to 4 mg/kg/day PO.
         d) Phenobarbital maintenance 2.5 mg/kg/dose given twice daily.
   c. Choreiform movement and grossly inadequate behavior are major neurologic complications. Phar-

macologic control is difficult. These complications usually but not always clear without demonstrable sequelae.

C. Management of Selected Complications

1. Chylothorax: Chylothorax, the accumulation of chyle in the pleural cavity, may be caused by cutting large tributaries of the thoracic duct. It may occur after repair of COA, Blalock-Taussig or Gore-Tex interposition shunt, or rarely after the repair of PDA. Chylothorax (with occasional chylopericardium) may result from the combination of transection of small lymph channels, and an elevated SVC pressure and may follow a Senning operation or SVC-RPA anastomosis (bidirectional Glenn operation).

   The fluid may or not have creamy appearance, but a triglyceride level above 110 mg/dl is highly probable of the diagnosis. When the patient ingests butter, the fluid usually becomes creamy. Infection of chylothorax has not been reported.

   Treatment is directed at drainage of chylothorax (chest tube placement) and reducing the flow of lymph (by limiting physical activity to reduce lymph flow from the extremities).

   a. In most cases chest tube drainage is all that is necessary. If chylothorax develops after chest tube removal, needle aspiration every 3 to 4 days usually constitutes adequate treatment. The drainage slows or stops within 7 days in most cases. Careful attention to the nutrition of the patient is important.

   b. Either parenteral hyperalimentation or a diet with medium-chain triglyceride as the fat source is called for; medium-chain triglycerides are absorbed by the portal system, not the lymphatic system.

   c. If the drainage is large or persists, surgical intervention may be considered. Indications for the intervention may include (1) average daily loss above 100 ml/age/day for 5 days, (2) the chyle flow not slowing after 2 weeks, or (3) imminent nutritional complications.

    d. Tetracycline pleurodesis has been used successfully.
    e. Pleuroperitoneal shunt has been suggested.
2. Persistent pleural effusion, which is common after a
   Fontan operation, creates a management problem. It
   results from the high right-sided venous pressure.
    a. Diuretics may be useful in treatment of the effu-
       sion.
    b. Catheter or chest tube drainage can be used to re-
       duce respiratory symptoms. When the drainage is
       large, appropriate replacement of fluid, electro-
       lytes, and protein is important.
    c. Pleurodesis with a sclerosing agent (e.g., tetracy-
       cline) may be effective.
    d. Pleuroperitoneal shunt may be considered.
3. Paralysis of the diaphragm occurs in about 1% of patients after thoracic surgery. It is the result of damage
   to the phrenic nerve. It may occur after PDA ligation,
   S-P shunt, or open heart surgery and may be due to
   nerve transection, blunt trauma, stretching during retraction, electrocautery, or hypothermic injury by
   ice slush used in open heart surgery. It is more common on the left side than on the right.
       The diagnosis should be suspected if there is persis-
   tent unexplained tachypnea, respiratory distress, hypoxia and/or hypercarbia, atelectasis, or inability to
   wean from the ventilator. CXR films are helpful if the
   patient is not on a ventilator. Echo is diagnostic if it is
   done during spontaneous breathing. When paralysis
   is not caused by transection, return of function usually occurs in 2 weeks to 6 months. Management
   ranges from conservative to surgical intervention.
    a. Some investigators recommend ventilator support
       only for the initial 2 to 6 weeks.
    b. Continuous positive airway pressure (CPAP) may
       be useful in management as well as in identifying
       patients who may benefit from plication.
    c. If respiratory insufficiency persists, surgical plica-
       tion should be considered. Plication of the dia-
       phragm usually is not necessary as long as the pa-

tient can be extubated without developing respiratory insufficiency.

III. POSTOPERATIVE SYNDROMES

Four well-recognized syndromes are seen in the period following open heart surgery in children.

A. Postcoarctectomy Hypertension

Paradoxic hypertension following coarctation surgery is quite common, with a mild degree of systolic hypertension developing within 36 hours after coarctation surgery, followed by a more delayed diastolic hypertension and lasting for 7 to 14 days. The sympathetic nervous system and the renin-angiotensin system are believed to be responsible for the hypertension. In about 10% to 20% of cases, mild abdominal discomfort and distention are noted during the first 5 or 6 postoperative days.

Postcoarctectomy syndrome, first described in the 1950s, is rare. Occurring in up to 5% of patients, it is characterized by severe, intermittent abdominal pain beginning 4 to 8 days after surgery with accompanying fever and leukocytosis. In severe cases abdominal distention, ileus, melena, and gangrenous bowel were reported. Persistent paradoxic hypertension may be present. Abdominal findings are believed to be caused by arteritis resulting from sudden increase in pulsatile pressures in arteries distal to the coarctation, and the hypertension may be due to an altered baroreceptor response plus an increased excretion of epinephrine or norepinephrine.

BP should be monitored carefully in the postoperative period to detect rebound hypertension. The hypertension in the arm may be due to a residual coarctation or an improper BP measuring technique rather than a generalized rebound hypertension. Feeding of solid foods is delayed in patients with postoperative coarctation. Reduction of rebound hypertension may be accomplished by (1) administration of a β-adrenergic blocker such as propranolol 0.01 to 0.05 mg/kg IV over 10 min every 6 to 8 hours,

(2) a vasodilator such as hydralazine or nitroprusside, (3) an ACE inhibitor such as captopril, or (4) a sympatholytic agent such as reserpine.

B. Postpericardiotomy Syndrome

Postpericardiotomy syndrome, a febrile illness with pericardial and pleural reaction, develops after surgery involving pericardiotomy. It is believed to be an autoimmune response in association with a recent or remote viral infection. Patients who develop the syndrome have a high titer of antiheart antibodies along with high antibody titers against adenovirus, coxsackievirus B1-6, and cytomegalovirus. This occurs in about 25% to 30% of patients who receive pericardiotomy.

Onset is a few weeks to a few months (median 4 weeks) after surgery that involves pericardiotomy. The syndrome is characterized by fever (sustained or spiking up to 40°C, or 104°F) and chest pain. Chest pain, which may be severe, is caused by both pericarditis and pleuritis. It is rare in infants less than 2 years of age. Physical examination usually reveals pericardial and pleural friction rubs and hepatomegaly. Tachycardia, tachypnea, rising venous pressure, and falling arterial pressure with a paradoxic pulse are signs of cardiac tamponade. CXR film shows enlarged cardiac silhouette and pleural effusion. The ECG shows persistent ST segment elevation and flat or inverted T waves in the limb and left precordial leads. Echo is the most reliable test in confirming the presence and amount of pericardial effusion and in evaluating evidence of cardiac tamponade. Leukocytosis with shift to the left and elevated erythrocyte sedimentation rate are present. While the disease is self-limiting, its duration is highly variable; the median duration is 2 to 3 weeks. Some 21% of patients have recurrences.

Bed rest is all that is needed for a mild case. A nonsteroidal antiinflammatory agent such as ibuprofen or indomethacin is effective in most cases. In severe cases moderate doses of corticosteroids for a few days may be indicated if the diagnosis is secure and infection has been ruled out. Emergency pericardiocentesis may be required if signs of cardiac tamponade are present. Diuretics may be used for pleural effusion.

C. Postperfusion Syndrome

Postperfusion syndrome, which occurs only after open heart surgery using a pump oxygenator, is caused by a cytomegalovirus infection. The virus is believed to be transmitted to the patient from an inapparent viremia of healthy donors. Postperfusion syndrome has almost disappeared since freshly drawn blood is no longer used, except in patients with severe cyanotic heart defects.

The onset is 4 to 6 weeks after a cardiac surgery with cardiopulmonary bypass. It is characterized by the triad of fever, splenomegaly, and atypical lymphocytosis. Hepatomegaly is also common. Fever is low grade, 38° to 39°C (100.4° to 102.2°F). Malaise and anorexia are common. The fever and atypical lymphocytosis have short duration (about 2 weeks), but splenomegaly usually lasts 3 to 4 weeks to 3 to 4 months. No recurrence has been reported. Cytomegalovirus may be demonstrated in the urine, or a changing titer to the virus may be demonstrated in the serum.

No specific treatment is available. The syndrome is self-limiting, lasting for weeks to a few months.

D. Hemolytic Anemia Syndrome

Hemolytic anemia may follow cardiac surgery, especially repair of endocardial cushion defect, other congenital heart defects using a synthetic patch material, or aortic or mitral valve replacement. Hemolysis is caused by unusual intracardiac turbulence.

The onset is 1 to 2 weeks after surgery with placement or insertion of synthetic and prosthetic materials. It is characterized by low-grade fever, anemia, jaundice, dark urine, hepatomegaly, and reticulocytosis. Iron deficiency anemia may develop because of excessive loss of iron in the urine in chronic disease. Peripheral smears reveal abnormal crenated and fragmented red blood cells and reticulocytosis. Hemoglobinemia, methemalbuminemia, and hemosiderinuria are also present.

Anemia is treated with either iron replacement therapy or blood transfusion. Most patients respond to oral iron therapy. Surgical correction of turbulence is indicated if the anemia is severe and the correction is technically possible.

CARDIOVASCULAR IX DRUG DOSAGE

Drug dosages listed in this chapter are derived primarily from the following sources.

1. *Physician's desk reference,* ed 49, Montvale, NJ, Medical Economics Data Production, 1995.
2. Benitz WE, Tatro DS: *The pediatric drug handbook,* ed 2, Chicago, Year Book Medical, 1988.
3. Johnson KB: *The Harriet Lane handbook,* ed 13, St. Louis, Mosby, 1993.
4. Levin RH, Zenk KE: Medication table. Rudolph AM, Hoffman JIE, Rudolph CM, editors: *Pediatrics,* ed 19, Norwalk, Appleton and Lange, 1991.

Formulary

Drug	Route and Dosage	Toxicity or Side Effects	How Supplied
Adenosine (Adenocard) (antiarrhythmic)	*Children and Adults:* (IV): 50 µg/kg Repeat q1-2 min, increasing to 250 µg/kg	Transient bradycardia and tachycardia, transient AV block in atrial flutter, fibrillation (±)	Inj: 3 mg/ml
Amiodarone (Cordarone) (class III antiarrhythmic agent)	*Children:* (PO): 5-10 mg/kg/day in 2 doses for 10 days. If responsive, 3-5 mg/kg once a day; may be reduced to 2.5 mg/kg for 5 of 7 days thereafter *Adults:* (PO): *Loading:* 800-1600 mg/day for 1-3 wk; then reduce to 600-800 mg/day for 1 mo *Maintenance:* 400 mg day	Progressive dyspnea and cough, worsening of arrhythmias, hepatotoxicity, nausea, vomiting, corneal microdeposits, hypotension, heart block, ataxia, hypothyroidism, hyperthyroidism, photosensitivity	Tab: 200 mg
Amrinone (Inocor) (noncatecholamine intropic agent with vasodilator effects)	*Children:* (IV): *Loading:* 0.5 mg/kg over 2-3 min in 1/2 NS (not D₅W) *Maintenance:* 5-20 µg/kg/min *Adults:* (IV): *Loading:* 0.75 mg/kg over 2-3 min *Maintenance:* 5-10 µg/kg/min	Thrombocytopenia, hypotension, tachyarrhythmias, hepatotoxicity, nausea, vomiting, fever	Inj: 5 mg/ml (20 ml)

Atenolol (Tenormin) (β_1-adrenoceptor blocker, antihypertensive, antiarrhythmic)	**Children:** (PO): 1-2 mg/kg/day **Adults:** (PO): 50 mg once a day for 1-2 wk (alone or with diuretic for hypertension) May increase to 100 mg once a day	CNS symptoms (dizziness, tiredness, depression), bradycardia, postural hypotension, nausea, vomiting, rash, blood dyscrasias (agranulocytosis, purpura)	Tab: 25, 50, 100 mg Inj: 0.5 mg/ml
Azathioprine (Imuran) (immunosuppressive agent)	**Children:** (PO): **Starting dose:** 2 mg/kg/day (to produce WBC count around 5000/mm³; may be reduced if WBC count falls below 4000/mm³	Leukopenia and/or thrombocytopenia; nausea, vomiting	Tab: 50 mg Inj: 5 mg/ml
Berylium tosylate (Bretylol) (class III antiarrhythmic agent)	**For ventricular fibrillation or tachycardia** **Children:** (IV): 5 mg/kg/dose over 8 min, then 10 mg/kg/dose q15-30 min (max 30 mg/kg) **Adults:** (IV): 5-10 mg/kg bolus over 8 min q6hr or 1-2 mg/min IV infusion	Hypotension, worsening of arrhythmias, aggravation of digitoxicity, nausea, vomiting	Inj: 50 mg/ml (10 ml ampule)
Captopril (Capoten) (ACE inhibitor, antihypertensive, vasodilator)	**Children:** (PO): Newborn: 0.1-1.4 mg/kg/dose 1-4 times day Infant: 0.5-0.6 mg/kg/day, in 1-4 doses	Neutropenia, agranulocytosis, proteinuria, hypotension, tachycardia, rash, taste impairment, small increase in serum potassium level (±)	Tab: 12.5, 25, 50, 100 mg

Continued.

Formulary—cont'd

Drug	Route and Dosage	Toxicity or Side Effects	How Supplied
	Child: 12.5 mg/dose 1-2 times/day (smaller dose in renal impairment)		
	Adults: (PO): 25 mg, 2-3 times/day initially Increase to usual dose of 50 mg 3 times/day for 1-2 wk Increase 25 mg/dose q1-2 wk to maximum 150 mg 3 times/day (Usually used with diuretic; smaller dose in renal impairment)		
Chloral hydrate (Notec) (sedative, hypnotic)	*Children:* **Sedative** (PO, PR): 25 mg/kg/dose q8h **Hypnotic** (PO, PR): 50-75 mg/kg/dose *Adults:* **Sedative** (PO, PR): 250 mg/dose 3 times/day	Mucous membrane irritation (layringospasm if aspirated), GI irritation, excitement/delirium (contraindicated in hepatic and renal impairment)	Syrup: 250, 500 mg/5 ml Supp: 324, 500, 648 mg

Drug	Dosage	Side effects	Supplied
Chlorothiazide (Diuril) (diuretic)	**Hypnotic** (PO, PR): 500-2000 mg/dose *Children:* (PO): 20-40 mg/kg/day in 2 doses *Adults:* (PO): 250-500 mg/dose once a day or intermittently	Hypokalemia, hyponatremia, hypochloremic alkalosis, prerenal azotemia, hyperuricemia, hyperglycemia, rarely blood dyscrasias, allergic reactions	PO susp: 250 mg/5 ml Tab: 250, 500 mg Inj: 500 mg (vial, for reconstruction with 18 ml sterile water)
Chlorpromazine (Thorazine) (sedative, antiemetic)	**For sedation or nausea** *Children >6 mo:* (IM): 0.5 mg/kg/dose q6-8h p.r.n. (PO): 0.5 mg/kg/dose q4-6h p.r.n. (PR): 1-2 mg/kg/dose q6-8h p.r.n. *Adults:* (IM): 25 mg test dose, then 25-50 mg q3-4h (PO): 10-25 mg q4-6h (PR): 100 mg q6-8h	Hypotension, arrhythmias, first-degree AV block, ST-T changes, hepatotoxicity, leukopenia or agranulocytosis	Inj: 25 mg/ml Syrup: 10 mg/5 ml (120 ml) Tab: 10, 25, 50, 100, 200 mg Supp: 25, 100 mg
Cholestyramine (Questran) (cholesterol-lowering agent)	*Children:* (PO): 250-1500 mg/kg/day in 2-4 doses *Adults:* (PO): *Starting dose:* 1 packet (or scoopful) of Questran Powder or Light 1-2 times/day	Constipation, other GI symptoms, hyperchloremic acidosis, bleeding	Packet of 9 g Questran Powder or 5 g Questran Light, each packet containing 4 g an-

Continued.

Formulary—cont'd

Drug	Route and Dosage	Toxicity or Side Effects	How Supplied
			hydrous cho-lestyramine resin
Clofibrate (Atromid-S) (antilipidemic, triglyceride lowering agent)	*Maintenance:* 2-4 packets or scoopfuls/day in 2 doses (or 1-6 doses) (max 6 packets/day) *Children:* (PO): 0.5-1.5 mg/day in 2-3 doses *Adults:* (PO): *Initial and maintenance:* 2 g/day in 2-3 doses	Nausea, other GI symptoms (vomiting, diarrhea, flatulence), headache, dizziness, fatigue, rash, blood dyscrasias, myalgia, arthralgia, hepatic dysfunction	Caps: 500 mg
Colestipol (Colestid) (lipid-lowering agent)	*Children:* (PO): 300-1500 mg/day in 2-4 doses *Adults:* (PO): *Starting dose:* 5 g 1-2 times/day; increment of 5 g q1-2 mo *Maintenance:* 5-30 g/day in 2-4 doses (Mix with 3-6 oz water or other fluid)	Constipation and other GI symptoms (abdominal distention, flatulence, nausea, vomiting, diarrhea), rarely rash, muscle and joint pain, headache, dizziness	Packet: 5 g

Cyclosporine (Sandimmune) (immunosuppressive agent)	*Children:* (PO): 5-10 mg/kg/day in 2-3 doses for 3 wks postop (blood level 300-400 ng/ml); then reduce to 4-6 mg/kg/day (blood level 100-200 ng/ml)	Nephrotoxicity, tremor, hypertension, less commonly hepatotoxicity, hirsutism, gum hypertrophy, rarely lymphoma, hypomagnesemia	Oral sol: 100 mg/ml Gelatin caps: 25, 100 mg
Diazepam (Valium) (sedative, anti-anxiety, anti-seizure agent)	*For sedation* *Children >6 mo:* (IM, IV): 0.1-0.3 mg/kg/dose q2-4h (max 0.6 mg/kg in 8 hr) (PO): 0.2-0.8 mg/kg/day in 3-4 doses, or 1-2.5 mg 3-4 times/day initially and increase p.r.n. *Adults:* (IM, IV): 2-10 mg/dose q3-4h p.r.n. (PO): 2-10 mg/dose q6-8h p.r.n.	Apnea, drowsiness, ataxia, rash, hypotension, bradycardia, hyperexcited state	Inj: 5 mg/ml Tab: 2, 5, 10 mg
Diazoxide (Hyperstat) (peripheral vasodilator)	*For emergency use only* *Children and Adults:* (IV): 1-3 mg/kg (max 150 mg single dose), repeat q5-15 min, titrate to desired effects	Hypotension, transient hyperglycemia, nausea, vomiting, sodium retention (CHF±)	Inj: 15 mg/ml
Digitoxin (Crystodigin, Purodigin) (cardiac glycoside)	*Children:* *TDD:* (PO): Premature and full-term newborn 20 μg/kg 1 mo-2yr 30 μg/kg >2yr 20 μg/kg	Same as for digoxin	Elixir: 50 μg/ml Tab: 0.05, 0.1 mg Inj: 0.2 mg/ml

Continued.

Formulary—cont'd

Drug	Route and Dosage	Toxicity or Side Effects	How Supplied
	(IV, IM): Same as PO TDD **Maintenance dose:** (PO, IV, IM): 15% (10%–20%) of TDD once a day **Adults:** (PO): **Loading:** 0.6 mg initially, then 0.4 mg, then 0.2 mg q4-6hr **Maintenance:** 0.15 mg once a day (ranges 0.05–0.3 mg/day)		
Digoxin Immune Fab (Digibind) (digoxin antidote)	**Infants and children:** (IV): 1 vial (40 mg) dissolved in 4 ml H$_2$O, over 30 min **Adults:** (IV): 4 vials (240 mg)	Hypokalemia, rapid AV conduction in atrial flutter, rarely allergic reaction	Vial: 40 mg
Digoxin (Lanoxin) (cardiac glycoside)	**Children:** TDD (PO): Premature 20 µg/kg Full-term newborn 30 µg/kg 1 mo-2yr 40-50 µg/kg 2 yr 30-40 µg/kg	AV conduction disturbances, arrhythmias, nausea and vomiting	Elixir: 50 µg/ml (60 ml) Tab: 0.125, 0.25, 0.5 mg Inj: 100, 250 µg/ml

Drug	Dosage	Side effects	Preparations
	(IV): 75%-80% of PO dose *Maintenance dose:* (PO): 25%-30% of TDD/day in 2 doses		Lanoxicaps: 0.05, 0.1, 0.2 mg
Disopyramide (Norpace) (class IA antiarrhythmic agent)	*Adults:* (PO): *Loading:* 8-12 µg/kg *Maintenance:* 0.10-0.25 mg/day *Children:* (PO): <1 yr: 10-30 mg/kg/day q6h 1-4 yr: 10-20 mg/kg/day q6h 4-12 yr: 10-15 mg/kg/day q6h 12-18 yr: 6-15 mg/kg/day q6h (q4h dosing when given regular caps) *Adults:* (PO): 600 mg/day (400-800 mg/day) in 4 doses of caps or 2 doses of controlled release (CR) caps. Initially use regular caps and later switch to CR caps (twice a day)	Heart failure, hypotension, anticholinergic effects (urinary retention, dry mouth, constipation), nausea, vomiting, hypoglycemia	Caps: 100, 150 mg CR caps: 100, 150 mg
Dobutamine (Dobutrex) (β₁-adrenergic stimulator)	*Children:* (IV): 2-15 µg/kg/min in D₅W or NS (incompatible with alkali solution)	Tachyarrhythmias, hypertension, nausea, vomiting, headache (contraindicated in IHSS and atrial flutter, fibrillation)	Inj: 12.5 mg/ml (20 ml vial)

Continued.

Formulary—cont'd

Drug	Route and Dosage	Toxicity or Side Effects	How Supplied
Dopamine (Intropin, Dopastat) (natural catecholamine, inotropic agent)	**Adults:** (IV): 2.5-10 μg/kg/min (max 40 μg/kg/min) **Children:** (IV): Effects are dose dependent: 2-5 μg/kg/min: ↑renal blood flow (RBF) and urine output 5-15 μg/kg/min: ↑RBF, ↑heart rate, ↑cardiac contractility, cardiac output 20 μg/kg/min: α-adrenergic effects with ↓RBF(±) (Incompatible with alkali solution)	Tachyarrhythmias, nausea, vomiting, hypotension or hypertension, extravasation (tissue necrosis: treat with local infiltration of phentolamine)	Inj: 40 mg/ml (5 ml), 80 mg/ml (5 ml), 160 mg/ml (5 ml)
Enalapril (Vasotec) (ACE inhibitor, vasodilator)	**Children:** (PO): 0.1 mg/kg once or twice daily (max 0.5 mg/kg/day) **Adults:** **For CHF** (PO): Start with 2.5 mg once or twice daily (usual range 5-20 mg/day)	Hypotension, dizziness, fatigue, headache	Tab: 2.5, 5, 10, 20 mg

Drug	Dosage	Adverse effects	How supplied
Ephedrine sulfate (α- and β-adrenoceptor stimulant)	**For hypertension** (PO): Start with 5 mg once a day (usual dose 10-40 mg/day) *Children:* (IV, IM): 0.2-0.3 mg/kg/dose q4-6h p.r.n. *Adults:* (IV): 5-25 mg/dose q3-4h (IM, SC): 25-50 mg/dose q4-6h		Inj: 25, 50 mg/ml
Epinephrine (Adrenalin) (α-, β$_1$-, β$_2$-adrenergic stimulator)	*Children:* (IV): 1:10,000 solution Begin with 0.1 µg/kg/min, increase to 1 µg/kg/min to achieve desired effects	Similar to epinephrine	Inj: 0.01 mg/ml (1:100,000 solution, 5 ml) 0.1 mg/ml (1:10,000 solution, 10 ml) 1 mg/ml (1:1,000 solution, 1 ml)
Ethacrynic acid (Edecrin) (loop diuretic)	*Children:* (PO): 25 mg/dose once a day (max 2-3 mg/kg/day) (IV): 1 mg/kg/dose *Adults:* (PO): 50-100 mg once a day (max 400 mg) (IV): 0.5-1 mg/kg/dose or 50 mg/dose	Tachyarrhythmias, hypertension, nausea, vomiting, headache, tissue necrosis (±) Dehydration, hypokalemia, prerenal azotemia, hyperuricemia, 8th cranial nerve damage (deafness), abnormal LFT, agranulocytosis or thrombocytopenia, GI irritation, rash	Tab: 25, 50 mg Inj: 50 mg (vial for reconstitution with 50 ml D$_5$W)

Continued.

Formulary—cont'd

Drug	Route and Dosage	Toxicity or Side Effects	How Supplied
Fentanyl (Sublimaze) (narcotic analgesic)	**For sedation** *Children:* (IV): 1-3 yr: 2-3 µg/kg/dose 3-12 yr: 1-2 µg/kg/dose >12 yr: 0.5-1.0 µg/kg/dose; may repeat q30-60min *Adults:* (IV): 50-100 µg/dose	Respiratory depression, apnea, rigidity, bradycardia	Inj: 50 µg/ml
Furosemide (Lasix) (loop diuretic)	*Children:* (IV): 0.5-2 mg/kg/dose 2-4 times/ day (PO): 1-2 mg/kg/dose 1-3 times/ day p.r.n. (max 6 mg/kg/dose) *Adults:* (IV): 20-40 mg/dose 2-4 times/ day (PO): 20-80 mg/dose 1-4 times/ day p.r.n.	Hypokalemia, hyperuricemia, prerenal azotemia, ototoxicity, rarely blood dyscrasias, rash	PO sol: 10 mg/ml (60 ml) Tab: 20, 40, 80 mg Inj: 10 mg/ml (2.4, 10 ml)
Heparin (anticoagulant)	*Children:* (IV): *Initial dose:* 50 U/kg IV injection *Maintenance:* 100 U/kg q4h	Bleeding (antidote protamine sulfate)	Inj: 1,000, 2,500, 5,000, 7,500, 10,000 U/ml

Drug	Dosage	Adverse effects	Supplied
Hydralazine (Apresoline) (peripheral vasodilator, antihypertensive)	(IV drip): 20,000 U/m²/24h Keep whole-blood clotting time 2.5-3 times control or APTT 1.5-2 times control *Adults:* (IV): *Initial dose:* 10,000 U IV injection *Maintenance:* 5000-10,000 U q4-6h (IV drip): Initial dose: 5000 U followed by 20,000-40,000 U/day *Children:* (IM, IV): 0.15-0.2 mg/kg/dose (for emergency) May be repeated q4-6h (PO): 0.75-3 mg/kg/day in 2-4 doses *Adults:* (IM, IV): 20-40 mg/kg/dose (for emergency), repeat p.r.n. (PO): Start with 10 mg 4 times/day for 3-4 days, increase to 25 mg 4 times/day for 3-4 days, then up to 50 mg 4 times/day	Hypotension, tachycardia and palpitation, lupuslike syndrome with prolonged use (fever, arthralgia, splenomegaly and +LE prep), blood dyscrasias	Inj: 20 mg/ml Tab: 10, 25, 50, 100 mg
Hydrochlorothiazide (HydroDiuril) (diuretic)	*Children:* (PO): 2-4 mg/kg/day in 2 doses	Same as for chlorothiazide	Tab: 25, 50, 100 mg

Continued.

Formulary—cont'd

Drug	Route and Dosage	Toxicity or Side Effects	How Supplied
Hydroxyzine (Vistaril, Atarax) (sedative)	*Adults:* (PO): 25-100 mg/day, single or divided doses May be given intermittently *Children:* (IM): 1 mg/kg/dose q4-6h p.r.n. (PO): <6 yr: 50 mg/day in 4 doses >6 yr: 50-100 mg/day in 4 doses	CNS symptoms (drowsiness, tremor, convulsion, anti-cholinergic effects (dry mouth, blurred vision, palpitation, hypotension, urinary frequency)	Inj: 25, 50 mg/ml PO susp: 25 mg/5 ml Tab: 10, 25, 50, 100 mg Caps: 25, 50, 100 mg
Indomethacin (Indocin) (prostaglandin synthesis inhibitor, non-steroidal anti-inflammatory)	*Adults:* (IM): 25-100 mg q4-6h (max 600 mg/day) (PO): 50-100 mg q6h **For PDA closure in premature infants** (IV): 0.2 mg/kg initially, then 0.1 mg/kg (for age <48 hr) 0.2 mg/kg (for age 2-7 days) 0.25 mg/kg (for age >7 days) May be given up to 2 doses, q12h (total up to 3 doses)	GI or other bleeding, GI disturbances, renal impairment, electrolyte disturbances ($\downarrow$Na, $\uparrow$K)	Vial: 1 mg
Isoproterenol (Isuprel) (β1-, β2-adrenergic stimulator)	*Children:* (IV): 0.1-0.5 µg/kg/min; titrate to desired effect	Similar to epinephrine	Inj: 0.2 mg/ml (1 : 5,000 solution: 1.5 ml)

Drug	Dosage		How supplied
Ketamine (Ketalar) (dissociate anesthetic)	*Adults:* (IV): 2-20 µg/min; titrate to desired effect (incompatible with alkali solution) *Children:* (IM): 8-12 mg/kg Repeat smaller doses q30min p.r.n. (IV): 2-3 mg/kg/dose Repeat smaller dose q30min p.r.n.	Hypertension, tachycardia, respiratory depression, apnea, CNS symptoms (dreamlike state, confusion, agitation)	Inj: 10, 50, 100 mg/ml
Lidocaine (Xylocaine) (class IB antiarrhythmic agent)	*Children:* (IV): *Loading:* 1 mg/kg/dose q5-10min p.r.n. *Maintenance:* 30 µg/kg/min IV drip (range 20-50 µg/kg/min) *Adults:* (IV): *Loading:* 1 mg/kg/dose q5min *Maintenance:* 1-4 mg/min IV drip	Seizure, respiratory depression, CNS symptoms (anxiety, euphoria, drowsiness), arrhythmias, hypotension, shock	Inj: 10 mg/ml (5 ml ampule), 20 mg/ml (5, 10 ml ampule)
Meperidine (Demerol) (narcotic analgesic)	*Children:* (IM, IV, PO): 1-1.5 mg/kg/dose q3-4h p.r.n. *Adults:* (IM, IV, PO): 50-100 mg/dose q3-4h p.r.n.	Respiratory depression, hypotension, bradycardia, nausea, vomiting	Inj: 25, 50, 75, 100 mg/ml Tab: 50, 100 mg Syrup: 50 mg/ 5 ml

Continued.

Formulary—cont'd

Drug	Route and Dosage	Toxicity or Side Effects	How Supplied
Metaraminol (Aramine) (α-, β-adrenoceptor stimulant)	*Children:* (IV): 0.01 mg/kg/dose IV bolus or 5 µg/kg/min IV infusion initially; titrate to desired effect *Adults:* (IV): 0.5-5 mg IV bolus q5-10min p.r.n. 1.4 µg/kg/min IV infusion	Similar to norepinephrine	Inj: 10 mg/ml
Methyldopa (Aldomet) (antihypertensive)	*Children:* (IV): 5-10 mg/kg/dose over 30-60 min, then 20-40 mg/kg/day in 4 doses (max 65 mg/kg/day or 3 g/day) (PO): 10 mg/kg/day in 2-4 doses May be increased or decreased (max 65 mg/kg/day or 3 g/day) *Adults:* (IV): 250-500 mg q6h (max 1 g q6h) (PO): 250 mg 2-3 times/day for 2 days May be increased or decreased q2days Usual dose 0.5-2 g/day in 2-4 doses (max 3 g/day)	Sedation, orthostatic hypotension and bradycardia, lupuslike syndrome, Coombs (+) hemolytic anemia and leukopenia, hepatitis/cirrhosis, colitis, impotence	Inj: 50 mg/ml PO susp: 250 mg/ml (16 oz) Tab: 125, 250, 500

Metoprolol (Lopressor) (β-adrenoceptor blocker)	*Children >2 yr:* (PO): 1-5 mg/kg/day in 2 doses *Adults:* (PO): 100 mg/day in 1-3 doses initially; may increase to 450 mg/ day in 2-3 doses Usual dose 100-450 mg/day (Usually used with hydrochlorothiazide 25-100 mg/day)	CNS symptoms (dizziness, tiredness, depression), bronchospasm, bradycardia, diarrhea, nausea, vomiting, abdominal pain	Tab: 50, 100 mg
Mexiletine (Mexitil) (class 1B antiarrhythmic agent)	*Children:* (PO): 6-8 mg/kg/day initially, then 2-5 mg/kg/dose q6-8h; increase 1-2 mg/kg/dose q2-3days to desired effect (with food or antacid) *Adults:* (PO): 200 mg q8h for 2-3 days Increase to 300-400 mg/q8h (Usual dose 200-300 mg q8h) Therapeutic level: 0.75-2.0 µg/mL	Nausea, vomiting, CNS symptoms (headache, dizziness, tremor, paresthesia, mood changes), rash, hepatic dysfunction (±)	Caps: 150, 200, 250 mg
Milrinone (Primacor) (phosphodiesterase inhibitor, noncatecholamine inotropic, vasodilator agent)	*Children:* (IV): *Loading:* 10-50 µg/kg over 10 min, then 0.1-1 µg/kg/min drip *Adults:* (IV): *Loading:* 50 µg/kg over 10 min, then 0.5 µg/kg/min drip (ranges 0.375-0.75 µg/kg/min)	Arrhythmias, hypotension, hypokalemia, thrombocytopenia	Inj: 1 mg/ml

Continued.

Formulary—cont'd

Drug	Route and Dosage	Toxicity or Side Effects	How Supplied
Minoxidil (Loniten) (peripheral vasodilator)	*Children <12 yr:* (PO): 0.2 mg/kg/day in 1-2 doses initially Increase 0.1-0.2 mg/kg/day q3d until desired effects achieved (Usual dose 0.25-1 mg/kg/day in 1-2 doses; max 50 mg/day) *Children >12 yr and adults:* (PO): 5 mg once a day initially May be increased to 10, 20, 40 mg in single or divided doses (Usual dose 10-40 mg/day in 1-2 doses; max 100 mg/day)	Reflex tachycardia, fluid retention (used with a β-blocker and diuretic), pericardial effusion, hypertrichosis, rarely blood dyscrasias (leukopenia, thrombocytopenia)	Tab: 2.5, 10 mg
Morphine sulfate (narcotic analgesic)	*Children:* (SC, IM, IV): 0.1-0.2 mg/kg/dose q2-4h (max 15 mg/dose) *Adults:* (SC, IM, IV): 2.5-20 mg/dose q2-6h p.r.n.	CNS depression, respiratory depression, nausea, vomiting, hypotension, bradycardia	Inj: 8, 10, 15 mg/ml
Naloxone (Narcan) (narcotic antagonist)	*Children:* (IM, IV): 5-10 μg/kg/dose q2-3min for 1-3 doses p.r.n. (may need 5-10 doses) *Adults:* (IM, IV): 0.4-2 mg/dose q2-3min for 1-3 doses p.r.n.	Ventricular arrhythmia, pulmonary edema (±), nausea, vomiting, seizure	Inj: 0.4, 10 mg/ml Neonatal Narcan: 0.02 mg/ml

Drug	Dosage	Side effects	Supplied
Nifedipine (Procardia, Adalat) (calcium channel blocker, coronary vasodilator)	*Children:* (for hypertrophic cardiomyopathy) (PO): 0.6-0.9 mg/kg/day in 3-4 doses *Adults:* (for angina) (PO): 10 mg 3 times/day initially Titrate up to 20 or 30 mg 3-4 times/day over 7-14 days Usual dose 10-20 mg 3 times/day (max 180 mg/day)	Hypotension, peripheral edema, CNS symptoms (headache, dizziness, weakness), nausea	Caps: 10 mg
Nitroglycerine (Nitro-Bid IV) (peripheral vasodilator)	*Children:* (IV): Start at 0.5-1.0 µg/kg/min Increase 1 µg/kg/min q20min to titrate to effect (max 6 µg/kg/min) (Dilute in D₅W or NS with fliral concentration <400 µg/ml_, light sensitive) *Adults:* (IV): Initial dose: 5 µg/min through infusion pump Increase 5 µg/min q3-5min until desired effects achieved	Hypotension, tachycardia, headache, nausea, vomiting	Inj: 5 mg/ml
Nitroprusside (Nipride) (peripheral vasodilator)	*Children:* (IV): 0.5-8 µg/kg/min, with BP monitoring	Hypotension, sweating, palpitation, nausea, vomiting, cyanide toxicity (metabolic aci-	Inj: 50 mg (vial for 2-3 ml D₅W)

Continued.

Formulary—cont'd

Drug	Route and Dosage	Toxicity or Side Effects	How Supplied
	Usual dose 2-3 µg/kg/min (Dilute stock solution [50 mg] in 250-2000 ml D₅W, light sensitive)	dosis the earliest and most reliable evidence: monitor thiocyanate level when used >48h and in renal failure	
Norepinephrine (Levophed, Levarterenol) (α-, β-adrenoceptor stimulant)	*Children:* (IV): 0.1 µg/kg/min initially; increase dose to attain desired effects *Adults:* (IV): Add 4 ml norepinephrine to 1 L D₅W, stat at 2-3 ml/min (8-12 µg/min) and adjust rate	Hypertension, bradycardia (reflex), arrhythmias, tissue necrosis (treat with phentolamine infiltration)	Inj: 1 mg/ml
Phentolamine (Regitine) (α-adrenocepto blocker)	*For pheochromocytoma* *Children:* (IM, IV): 0.05-0.1 mg/kg/dose Repeat q5min until hypertension is controlled, then q2-4h p.r.n. *Adults:* (IM, IV): 2.5-5 mg/dose Repeat q5min until hypertension is controlled, then q2-4h p.r.n.	Hypotension, tachycardia, arrhythmias, nausea, vomiting	Inj: 5 mg/ml

Drug	Dosage	Adverse effects	Formulations
Phenylephrine (Neo-Synephrine) (α-adrenoceptor stimulant)	**For treatment of extravasated adrenergic drugs** (SC): 0.1-0.2 mg/kg locally within 12 hr (max 10 mg) **For hypotension** *Children:* (IM, SC): 0.1 mg/kg/dose q1-2h p.r.n. (IV): 5-10 µg/kg/dose IV bolus q10-15min or 0.1-0.5 µg/kg/min IV infusion *Adults:* (IM, SC): 2-5 mg/dose q1-2h p.r.n. (IV): 0.1-0.5 mg/dose IV bolus q10-15min p.r.n. Start IV infusion at 100-180 µg/min; maintain at 40-60 µg/min	Arrhythmias, hypertension, angina	Inj: 10 mg/ml
Phenytoin (Dilantin) (class IB antiarrhythmic agent)	*Children:* (IV): 2-4 mg/kg/dose over 5-10 min Followed by (PO): 2-5 mg/kg/day in 2-3 doses (Therapeutic level: 5-18 µg/ml for arrhythmias, 10-20 µg/ml for seizure)	Rash, Stevens-Johnson syndrome, CNS symptoms (ataxia, dysarthria), lupuslike syndrome, blood dyscrasias, peripheral neuropathy, gingival hypertrophy	Inj: 50 mg/ml PO susp: 30, 125 mg/5 mL (240 ml) Infatab: 50 mg (chewable) Caps: 30, 100 mg

Continued.

Formulary—cont'd

Drug	Route and Dosage	Toxicity or Side Effects	How Supplied
Potassium chloride	*Adults:* (IV): 100 mg q5min (total 500 mg) (PO): 250 mg 4 times for 1 day, 250 mg twice for 2 days, and 300-400 mg/day in 1-4 doses **Supplement in diuretic therapy** *Children:* (PO): 1-2 mEq/kg/day in 3-4 doses or 0.8-1.5 ml 10% KCl/kg/day 0.4-0.7 ml 20% KCl/kg/day in 3-4 doses	GI disturbances, ulcerations, hyperkalemia	10% sol: 1.3 mEq/ml 20% sol: 2.7 mEq/ml
Potassium gluconate	**Supplement in diuretic therapy** *Children:* (PO): 1-2 mEq/kg/day in 3-4 doses or 0.8-1.5 ml/kg/day in 3-4 doses	Same as for potassium chloride	Elixir: 1.3 mEq/ml
Potassium triplex (acetate-bicarbon-ate-citrate)	**Supplement in diuretic therapy** *Children:* (PO): 1-2 mEq/kg/day in 3-4 doses or 0.3-0.6 ml/kg/day in 3-4 doses	Same as for potassium chloride	PO sol: 3 mEq/ml

Prazosin (Minipress) (postsynaptic α-adrenergic blocker, antihypertensive)	**Children:** (PO): 5 µg/kg as a test dose, then 25-150 µg/kg/day in 4 doses **Adults:** (PO): 1 mg 2-3 times/day initially Increase to 20 mg/day in 2-4 doses Usual dose 6-15 mg/day	CNS symptoms (dizziness, headache, drowsiness), palpitation, nausea	Caps: 1, 2, 5 mg
Procaine amide (Pronestyl) (class IA antiarrhythmic agent)	**Children:** (IV): **Loading:** 3-6 mg/kg/dose over 5 min, repeated q10-30min (max 100 mg) **Maintenance:** 20-80 µg/kg/min by IV infusion (max 2 g/24 hr) (PO): 15-50 mg/kg/day q3-6h (max 4 g/24 hr) **Adults:** (IV): **Loading:** 50-100 mg/dose q5min p.r.n. **Maintenance:** 1-6 mg/min by IV infusion (PO): 250-500 mg/dose q3-6h (usual dose: 2-4 g/day) Therapeutic level: 4-10 µg/ml	Nausea, vomiting, blood dyscrasias, rash, lupuslike syndrome, hypotension, confusion, disorientation	Inj: 100, 500 mg/ml Tab: 250, 375, 500 mg Tab, sustained release: 250, 500 mg Caps: 250, 375, 500 mg

Continued.

Formulary—cont'd

Drug	Route and Dosage	Toxicity or Side Effects	How Supplied
Promethazine (Phenergan) (antiemetic)	**For nausea and vomiting** *Children:* (IM, PR): 0.25-0.5 mg/kg q4-6h p.r.n. *Adults:* (IM, PR): 12.5-25 mg q6h p.r.n. **For sedation before surgery** *Children:* (IM, PO, PR): 0.5-1 mg/kg/dose q6h p.r.n. *Adults:* (IM, PO, PR): 25-50 mg q4-6h p.r.n.	CNS stimulation, anticholinergic effects	Inj: 25, 50 mg/ml Tab: 12.5, 25, 50 mg Syrup: 6.25 mg/ 5 ml Supp: 12.5, 25, 50 mg
Propranolol (Inderal) (β-adrenoceptor blocker, class II antiarrhythmic agent)	**For hypertension** *Children:* (PO): 2-4 mg/kg/day in 2-4 doses (max 16 mg/kg/day) **For arrhythmias** *Children:* (IV): 0.01-0.15 mg/kg/dose over 10 min (max 1 mg/dose)	Hypotension, syncope, bronchospasm, nausea, vomiting, hypoglycemia, lethargy or depression, heart block	Tab: 10, 20, 40, 60, 80, 90 mg

Drug	Dosage	Side effects	Preparations
	(PO): 2-4 mg/kg/day in 3-4 doses (max 16 mg/kg/day)		
Prostaglandin E₁ (Prostin VR, Alprostadil)	*Adults:* (IV): 1 mg/dose q5 min (max 5 mg) (PO): 40-320 mg/day in 3-4 doses **For patency of ductus arteriosus** (IV): Begin infusion at 0.05-0.1 µg/kg/min When desired effect achieved, reduce to 0.05, 0.025, and 0.01 µg/kg/min If unresponsive, dose may be increased to 0.4 µg/kg/min	Apnea, flushing, bradycardia, hypotension, fever	Amp: 500 µg
Protamine sulfate	**Antidote to heparin overdose** (IV): Each 1 mg protamine neutralizes approximately 100 U heparin given in preceding 3-4 hr Slow IV infusion at a rate not exceeding 20 mg/min or 50 mg in any 10 min Check APTT	Hypotension, bradycardia, dyspnea, flushing, coagulation problem	Inj: 10 mg/ml
Quinidine gluconate (class IA antiarrhythmic agent)	*Children:* (PO): Test for idiosyncrasy with 2 mg/kg, 10-30 mg/kg/day in 2-3 doses Usual dose 160-660 mg q12h	Nausea, vomiting, ventricular arrhythmias, prolonged QRS, depressed myocardial contractility, blood dyscrasias, symptoms of cinchonism	Tab, sustained release: 330 mg Inj: 80 mg/ml

Continued.

Formulary—cont'd

Drug	Route and Dosage	Toxicity or Side Effects	How Supplied
Quinidine sulfate (class IA antiarrhythmic agent)	*Adults:* (PO): 25 mg test dose 200-400 mg q4-6h *Children:* (PO): Start with 3-6 mg/kg q2-3h for 5 doses May increase to 12 mg/kg q2-3h for 5 doses *Maintenance:* 7-12 mg/kg/day in 4 doses	Same as for quinidine gluconate	Caps: 200, 300 mg Tab: 100, 200, 300 mg Tab, sustained release: 300 mg
Reserpine (Serpasil) (depletion of NE store, antihypertensive)	*Children:* *For acute hypertension* (IM): 0.02-0.07 mg/kg q8-24h (max 2.5 mg/day) (may be used with hydralazine) (PO): 0.02 mg/kg/day in 2 doses *Adults:* (PO): 0.5 mg/day in 2 doses for 1-2 wk *Maintenance:* 0.1-0.25 mg/day	Mental depression, nasal stuffiness, bradycardia, hypotension	Inj: 2.5 mg/ml Tab: 0.1, 0.25 mg

Drug	Indication/Dosage	Notes	Supplied
Sodium polystyrene sulfonate (Kayexalate) (potassium lowering agent)	**For hyperkalemia** (slowly effective, taking hours to days) **Children:** (PO, NG): 1 g/kg/dose q6h (PR): 1 g/kg/dose q2-6h **Adults:** (PO, NG, PR): 15 g (4 level tsp) 1-4 times/day	(Cation exchange resin with practical exchange rates of 1 mEq K/1 g resin) NOTE: Delivers 1 mEq Na for each mEq K removed Nausea, vomiting, constipation, severe hypokalemia (monitor serum K, ECG, muscle weakness, confusion), hypocalcemia or hypernatremia (edema)	Powder: 454 g/lb Susp: 15 g/60 ml
Spironolactone (Aldactone) (aldosterone antagonist)	**Children:** (PO): 3 mg/kg/day in 1-3 doses **Adults:** (PO): 50-100 mg/day in 1-3 doses (max 200 mg/day)	Hyperkalemia (when given with potassium supplements), gynecomastia, agranulocytosis	Tab: 25, 50, 100 mg
Streptokinase (Streptase) (thrombolytic agent)	**Children:** (IV): **Loading:** 10,000 U/kg over 20-30 min (max 250,000 U) **Maintenance:** 1000 U/kg/hr in NS Obtain fibrinogen level in 4 hr (normal 2-4 g/L) Fibrinogen 1-1.4 g/L indicates effectiveness of therapy If no decrease in 4 hr, increase to 2000 U/kg hr in 500 U/kg/hr increments	Potential for allergic reaction with repeated use; premedicate with acetaminophen and antihistamine and repeat q4-6h	Inj: 250,000, 750,000, 1.5 million U/6.5 ml vial

Continued.

Formulary—cont'd

Drug	Route and Dosage	Toxicity or Side Effects	How Supplied
	If no decrease in fibrinogen level, switch to urokinase		
	Adults:		
	(IV): *Loading dose:* 250,000 U over 30 min		
	Maintenance: 100,000 U/hr for 24-72 hr		
	Obtain the following tests at baseline and q4h: APTT, TT, fibrinogen, PT, hematocrit, platelet count; APTT and TT should be <2 times control		
Tocainide (Tonocard) (class IB antiarrhythmic agent)	*Children:* (PO): 20-40 mg/kg/day in 3 doses	Dizziness, vertigo, nausea, vomiting, blood dyscrasias (±)	Tab: 400, 600 mg
	Adults: (PO): 400 mg q8h May increase to 600 mg q8h Usual dose 400-600 mg q8h		
Tolazoline (Priscoline) (α-adrenoceptor blocker)	*For neonatal pulmonary hypertension* (IV): *Loading:* 1-2 mg/kg over 10 min *Maintenance:* 1-2 mg/kg hr IV infusion	Hypotension and tachycardia, pulmonary hemorrhage, GI bleeding, arrhythmias, thrombocytopenia, leukopenia	Inj: 25 mg/ml

| Triamterene (Dyrenium) (potassium-conserving diuretic) | *Children:* (PO): 2-4 mg/kg/day in 1-2 doses *Adults:* (PO): 100-300 mg/day in 1-2 doses (max 300 mg) | Nausea, vomiting, leg cramps, dizziness, hyperuricemia, rash, prenal azotemia | Caps: 50, 100 mg |
| Urokinase (Abbokinase) (thrombolytic agent) | *Children:* **For clot lysis** (IV): *Loading:* 4000 U/kg/dose IV over 10 min *Maintenance:* 4000-6000 U/kg/hr (continue until the clot is dissolved, usually 24-72 hr) Monitor same lab tests as for streptokinase **For catheter clearance** (IV): Infuse 1 ml (containing 5000 U/ml) into catheter, aspirate with 5 ml syringe q5min 6 times May repeat urkinase infusion p.r.n. *Adults:* **For pulmonary embolism** (IV): *Priming dose:* 4400 U/kg 4400 U/kg/hr IV infusion for 12 hr by infusion pump | Bleeding, allergic reactions, rash, fever, chills, bronchospasm | Inj: 250,000 U/vial |

Continued.

Formulary—cont'd

Drug	Route and Dosage	Toxicity or Side Effects	How Supplied
Verapamil (Isoptin, Calan) (class IV antiarrhythmic agent)	*Children:* (IV): Child 0-1 yr: 0.1-0.2 mg/kg over 2 min Usual single dose 0.75-2 mg May repeat same dose in 30 min (should be used with extreme caution, only when other drugs fail) Child 1-15 yr: 0.1 mg/kg over 2 min (single max dose 2-5 mg) May repeat same dose in 15 min (PO): 35 mg/kg/day in 3 doses *Adults:* (IV): 5-10 mg over 2 min May repeat 10 mg in 30 min p.r.n. (PO): 240-480 mg/day in 3 doses	Hypotension, bradycardia, cardiac depression	Inj: 2.5 mg/ml Tab: 40, 80, 120 mg
Vitamin K	**Antidote to dicumarol or warfarin** (PO): 2.5-10 mg in 1 dose for correction of excessive PT from dicumarol or warfarin overdose		Tab: 5 mg

Warfarin (Coumadin)
(anticoagulant)

Children:
(PO): *Initial dose:* 1-3 mg q.d. for 2-4 days in evening (large loading dose not recommended)
Daily PT determination
Maintenance: 1-5 mg once a day
Keep INR 2.5-3.5
Heparin preferred initially for rapid anticoagulation; warfarin may be started concomitantly with heparin or may be delayed 3-6 days

Adults:
(PO): *Initial dose:* 2-5 mg q.d. for 2-4 days (large loading dose not recommended)
Adjust dosage to INR
Maintenance: 2-10 mg q.d.

Bleeding (Antidote: vitamin K, or fresh-frozen plasma)
Increased PT response
Salicylates, acetaminophen, alcohol, lipid-lowering agents, phenytoin, ibuprophen, some antibiotics
Decreased PT response
Antihistamines, barbiturates, oral contraceptives, vitamin C, high vitamin K diet

Tab: 1, 2, 2.5, 5, 7.5, 10 mg

ACE, angiotensin-converting enzyme; APTT, activated partial thromboplastin time; CHF, congestive heart failure; CNS, central nervous system; GI, gastrointestinal; INR, international normalized ratio; IV, intravenous; LFT, liver function test; NG, nasogastric; NS, normal saline; PO, by mouth; PR, per rectum; p.r.n., as needed; q, every; RBF, renal blood flow; SC, subcutaneous; TDD, total digitalizing dose; TT, thrombin time; WBC, white blood cell.

APPENDIX

FIG. A-1.
Antibiotic prophylaxis against bacterial endocarditis. (From Dajani AS et al: Prevention of bacterial endocarditis: recommendation by the American Heart Association, JAMA 264:2919-2922, 1990.)

Kilogram to pound conversion chart: (1 kg = 2.2 lb)

Kg	Lb
5	11.0
10	22.0
20	44.0
30	66.0
40	88.0
50	110.0

B. For patients considered to be at high risk who are not candidates for the standard regimen:

Ampicillin 2 g IV (or IM) plus gentamicin 1.5 mg/kg IV (or IM) (not to exceed 80 mg) 30 min before procedure, followed by amoxicillin 1.5 g orally 6 hours after the initial dose. Alternatively, the parenteral regimen may be repeated 8 hours after the initial dose.*

For amoxicillin/ampicillin/penicillin-allergic patients considered to be at high risk:

Vancomycin 1 g IV administered over 1 hour, starting one hour before the procedure. No repeat dose is necessary.*

*Note: Initial pediatric dosages are listed below. Follow-up oral dose should be one-half the initial dose. Total pediatric dose should not exceed total adult dose:

Amoxicillin:†	50 mg/kg	Vancomycin:	20 mg/kg
Clindamycin:	10 mg/kg	Ampicillin:	50 mg/kg
Erythromycin ethylsuccinate or stearate:	20 mg/kg	Gentamicin:	2.0 mg/kg

† The following weight ranges may also be used for the initial pediatric dose of amoxicillin:
<15 kg (33 lb), 750 mg
15-30 kg (33-66 lb), 1500 mg
>30 kg (66 lb), 3000 mg (full adult dose)

Name: _____

needs protection from
BACTERIAL ENDOCARDITIS
because of an existing
HEART CONDITION

Diagnosis: _____
Prescribed by: _____
Date: _____

For Dental/Oral/Upper Respiratory Tract Procedures

I. Standard Regimen in Patients at Risk (includes those with prosthetic heart valves and other high risk patients):

Amoxicillin 3 g orally 1 hour before procedure, then 1.5 g 6 hours after initial dose.*

For amoxicillin/penicillin-allergic patients:

Erythromycin ethylsuccinate 800 mg or erythromycin stearate 1 g orally 2 hours before a procedure, then one-half the dose 6 hours after the initial administration.*

—OR—

Clindamycin 300 mg orally 1 hour before a procedure and 150 mg 6 hours after initial dose.*

II. Alternative Prophylactic Regimens for Dental/Oral/Upper Respiratory Tract Procedures in Patients at Risk:

A. For patients unable to take oral medications:

Ampicillin 2 g IV (or IM) 30 min before procedure, then ampicillin 1 g IV (or IM) OR amoxicillin 1.5 g orally 6 hours after initial dose.*

—OR—

For ampicillin/amoxicillin/penicillin-allergic patients unable to take oral medications:

Clindamycin 300 mg IV 30 min before a procedure and 150 mg IV (or orally) 6 hours after initial dose.*

FIG A-1. For legend see opposite page.

For Genitourinary/Gastrointestinal Procedures

I. Standard regimen:

Ampicillin 2 g IV (or IM) plus gentamicin 1.5 mg/kg IV (or IM) (not to exceed 80 mg) 30 min before procedure, followed by amoxicillin 1.5 g orally 6 hours after the initial dose. Alternatively, the parenteral regimen may be repeated once 8 hours after the initial dose.*

For amoxicillin/ampicillin/penicillin-allergic patients:

Vancomycin 1 g IV administered over 1 hour plus gentamicin 1.5 mg/kg IV (or IM) (not to exceed 80 mg) 1 hour before the procedure. May be repeated once 8 hours after initial dose.**

II. Alternative oral regimen for low-risk patients:

Amoxicillin 3 g orally 1 hour before the procedure, then 1.5 g 6 hours after the initial dose.***

**Note: Initial pediatric dosages are listed below. Follow-up oral dose should be one-half the initial dose. Total pediatric dose should not exceed total adult dose.

Ampicillin:	50 mg/kg	Gentamicin:	2 mg/kg
Amoxicillin:	50 mg/kg	Vancomycin:	20 mg/kg

Note: Antibiotic regimens used to prevent recurrences of acute rheumatic fever are inadequate for the prevention of bacterial endocarditis. In patients with markedly compromised renal function, it may be necessary to modify or omit the second dose of gentamicin or vancomycin. Intramuscular injections may be contraindicated in patients receiving anticoagulants.

Adapted from *Prevention of Bacterial Endocarditis: Recommendations by the American Heart Association* by the Committee on Rheumatic Fever, Endocarditis, and Kawasaki Disease. *JAMA* 1990;264:2919–2922, © 1990 American Medical Association (also excerpted in *J Am Dent Assoc* 1991; 122:87–92).

Please refer to these joint American Heart Association–American Dental Association recommendations for more complete information as to which patients and which procedures require prophylaxis.

❤ American Heart Association

National Center
7320 Greenville Avenue
Dallas, Texas 75231

78-1003 (CP)
90-100M
4-91-511.2M
90 06 19 B

FIG. A-1, cont'd.

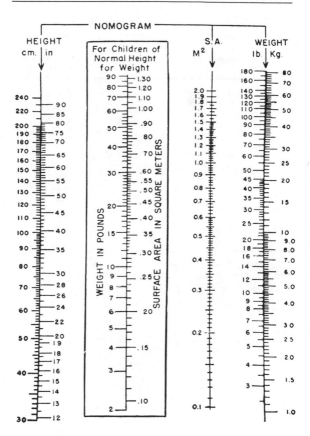

FIG. A-2.
Body surface nomogram.

TABLE A-1.

Recurrence Risks Given One Sibling Who Has a Cardiovascular Anomaly

Anomaly	Suggested Risk
Ventricular septal defect	3.0%
Patent ductus arteriosus	3.0
Atrial septal defect	2.5
Tetralogy of Fallot	2.5
Pulmonary stenosis	2.0
Coarctation of the aorta	2.0
Aortic stenosis	2.0
Transposition of the great arteries	1.5
AV canal (complete ECD)	2.0
Endocardial fibroelastosis	4.0
Triscupid atresia	1.0
Ebstein anomaly	1.0
Persistent truncus arteriosus	1.0
Pulmonary atresia	1.0
Hypoplastic left heart syndrome	2.0

Adapted from Nora JJ, Nora AH: The evaluation of specific genetic and environmental counseling in congenital heart diseases. Circulation *57:205-213, 1978.*

TABLE A-2.

Affected Offspring, Given One Parent with a Congenital Heart Defect

Defect	Mother Affected	Father Affected
Aortic stenosis	13-18%	3.%
Atrial septal defect	4-4.5	1.5
AV canal (Complete ECD)	14	1
Coarctation of the aorta	4	2
Patent ductus arteriosus	3.5-4	2.5
Pulmonary stenosis	4-6.5	2
Tetralogy of Fallot	6-10	1.5
Ventricular septal defect	6	2

From Nora JJ, Nora AH: Maternal transmission of congenital heart disease: new recurrence risk figures and the questions of cytoplasmic inheritance and vulnerability to teratogens. Am J Cardiol *59:459-463, 1987.*

TABLE A-3.

Normal M-Mode Echo Measurements (mm): Mean (95% prediction interval)

BW (kg)	3	5	8	10	15	20	25	30	40	50	60	70
BSA (m²)	0.24	0.34	0.45	0.52	0.68	0.82	0.94	1.06	1.27	1.47	1.65	1.82
IVS	4.5	4.5	5	5.5	6	7	7	7.5	8.5	8.5	9	9.5
	(3.5-5)	(4.5-5.5)	(4.5-6)	(4.5-6.5)	(5-7)	(5.5-8.5)	(5.5-9)	(6-9)	(6.5-10)	(7-10)	(8-10.5)	(7.5-11)
LVPW	4	4.5	5	5	6	6.5	7	7	8	8.5	8.5	9
	(3.5-5.5)	(4.5-5)	(4.5-6)	(4.5-6)	(5-7)	(5.5-8)	(6-8)	(6-8.5)	(6.5-9)	(7-9.5)	(7.5-10)	(7.5-11)
AO	12	13	15	16	18	19	21	22	23	25	26	27
	(10-14)	(11-16)	(12-17)	(13-18)	(15-22)	(16-23)	(17-24)	(18-26)	(19-27)	(20-29)	(21-30)	(23-32)
LA	18	20	21	22	25	27	28	30	32	33	34	36
	(15-21)	(16-23)	(17-25)	(18-26)	(21-29)	(22-32)	(23-33)	(24-35)	(26-37)	(27-38)	(28-41)	(29-42)
LVDD	21	25	28	29	33	35	37	39	42	44	46	48
	(18-23)	(22-27)	(24-31)	(25-32)	(29-36)	(31-39)	(33-41)	(34-43)	(37-47)	(39-49)	(41-51)	(42-53)
LVSD	14	16	17	18	21	23	24	25	27	28	29	31
	(12-17)	(13-19)	(14-21)	(15-22)	(17-24)	(18-27)	(19-28)	(21-29)	(22-32)	(23-33)	(24-34)	(25-36)

Adapted from data presented in graphic form by Henry WL, Ware J, Gardin JM, et al: Circulation 57:278-285, 1987. Values rounded off to the nearest 0.5 mm for IVS and LVPW and to the nearest 1 mm all other measurements. AO, aorta; BSA, body surface area; BW, body weight; IVS, interventricular septum; LA, left atrium; LVDD, left ventricular diastolic dimension; LVPW, left ventricular posterior wall; LVSD, left ventricular systolic dimension.

TABLE A-4.

Other Normal M-Mode Echo Values: Mean (95% CI)

LA/Ao ratio	1.1	(0.7-1.6)
IVS/LVPW ratio	1.1	(0.8-1.5)
FS = (LVDD − LVSD)/LVDD	0.36	(0.28-0.44)
EF = $(LVDD)^3 - (LVSD)^3/(LVDD)^3 \times 100$	74%	(64%-83%)
LPEP/LVET	0.35	(0.30-0.39)
RPEP/RVET	0.24	(0.16-0.30)

LA, left atrium; Ao, aorta; IVS, interventricular septum; LVPW, left ventricular posterior wall; FS, fractional shortening; EF, ejection fraction; LVDD, left ventricular diastolic dimension; LVSD, left ventricular systolic dimension; L(R)PEP, left (right) preejection period; LV(RV)ET, left (right) ventricular ejection time.

TABLE A-5.

Dimensions of Aorta and Pulmonary Arteries by 2D Echo

Echo Views	BSA (m²) BW (kg)	0.25 3	0.3 4	0.4 7	0.5 10
	Ascending aorta	10 (7-13)	11 (7.5-15)	13 (9-16)	14 (10-18)
	MPA	9 (5-12)	10 (6-13)	11 (7-14)	12 (8-16)
	RPA	5.5 (3.5-8)	6 (4-8.5)	6.5 (4.5-9)	7.5 (5-10)
	Ascending aorta	7.5 (4-10)	8 (4.5-11)	9 (6-12)	10 (6.5-13)
	Transverse aorta	6 (4-8.5)	7 (4.5-9)	8 (5.5-11)	9 (6.5-11)
	RPA	6 (4-8)	6.5 (4.5-9)	7.5 (5-10)	8.5 (6-11)
	Transverse aorta	9 (6-11)	10 (7-12.5)	11 (8-14)	12 (9.5-15)
	RPA	6 (4-8)	6.5 (4.5-9)	7 (5-10)	8 (6-10)

Adapted from data presented in graphic form by Snider AR, Enderlein MA, Teitel DF, et al: Am J Cardiol 53:218-224, 1984.
Values rounded off to the nearest 0.5 mm for measurements <10 mm and to the nearest 1 mm for measurements ≥10 mm. Figures in parentheses are tolerance limits weighted for BSA for prediction of

0.6	0.7	0.8	0.9	1.0	1.2	1.4
13	16	19	23	28	37	46

15	16	17	17	18	20	22
(11-19)	(12-20)	(12-21)	(13-22)	(14-23)	(15-25)	(16-27)
13	14	15	15	16	17	19
(9-17)	(9-18)	(11-19)	(11-20)	(12-21)	(13-23)	(14-24)
8	8.5	9	9	10	10	11
(5.5-10)	(6-11)	(7-11)	(7-12)	(7-12)	(8-14)	(8-15)
11	12	12	13	14	15	17
(7.5-14)	(8.5-15)	(9-16)	(9.5-13)	(11-18)	(12-19)	(14-21)
10	11	11	12	13	14	15
(7.5-12)	(8-13)	(8.5-14)	(9.5-15)	(10-16)	(11-17)	(12-18)
9	9.5	10	11	12	13	14
(6.5-11)	(7-12)	(8-13)	(9-14)	(9-15)	(10-16)	(11-17)
13	14	15	16	17	19	20
(10.5-16)	(11-17)	(13-18)	(13-20)	(14-20)	(15-22)	(17-24)
9	9.5	10	11	11	12	13
(6.5-11)	(7.5-11)	(8-12)	(9-13)	(9-14)	(10-15)	(11-16)

normal values for 80% of future population with 50% confidence. Measurements are made at end-diastolic (Q wave) using leading-edge technique.
BSA, body surface area; BW, body weight.

TABLE A-6.

Mitral and Tricuspid Valve Annulus Diameter by 2D Echo: Mean (95% CI)

BSA (m²) BW (kg)	0.2 2	0.25 3	0.3 4	0.4 7	0.5 10	0.6 13	0.7 16	0.8 19	0.9 23	1.0 28	1.2 37	1.4 46
Mitral valve (PL)	10 (7-13)	12 (9-15)	13 (10-16)	16 (13-19)	18 (15-21)	19 (16-23)	21 (18-24)	22 (18-26)	23 (19-26)	24 (20-27)	25 (22-28)	26 (23-30)
Mitral valve (A4C, S4C)*	12 (7-17)	15 (10-20)	17 (12-22)	20 (16-25)	23 (18-28)	25 (20-31)	27 (22-32)	29 (23-35)	31 (25-36)	32 (26-37)	35 (28-40)	36 (31-42)
Tricuspid valve (A4C, S4C)*	12 (8-17)	15 (10-19)	17 (12-22)	21 (16-26)	23 (18-29)	26 (20-31)	27 (22-33)	29 (23-36)	31 (24-37)	32 (25-38)	34 (27-42)	36 (28-44)

Adapted from data presented in graphic form by King DH, Smith EO, Huhta JC, et al: Am J Cardiol 55:787-789, 1985.

Measurements made at onset of R wave on ECG, using inner edge-to-inner edge method.

*Measurements greater of two projections; A4C amd S4C.

A4C, apical four-chamber view; S4C, subcostal four-chamber view; PL, parasternal long-axis view.

TABLE A-7.

Oxygen Consumption per Body Surface Area (ml/min/m^2) by Sex, Age, and Heart Rate

	Heart Rate (beats/min)												
Age (yr)	50	60	70	80	90	100	110	120	130	140	150	160	170
Male patients													
3				155	159	163	167	171	175	178	182	186	190
4			149	152	156	160	163	168	171	175	179	182	186
6		141	144	148	151	155	159	162	167	171	174	178	181
8		136	141	145	148	152	156	159	163	167	171	175	178
10	130	134	139	142	146	149	153	157	160	165	169	172	176
12	128	132	136	140	144	147	151	155	158	162	167	170	174
14	127	130	134	137	142	146	149	153	157	160	165	169	172
16	125	129	132	136	141	144	148	152	155	159	162	167	
18	124	127	131	135	139	143	147	150	154	157	161	166	
20	123	126	130	134	137	142	145	149	153	156	160	165	
25	120	124	127	131	135	139	143	147	150	154	157		
30	118	122	125	129	133	136	141	145	148	152	155		
35	116	120	124	127	131	135	139	143	147	150			
40	115	119	122	126	130	133	137	141	145	149			

Continued.

TABLE A-7.

Oxygen Consumption per Body Surface Area (ml/min/m²) by Sex, Age, and Heart Rate—cont'd

Age (yr)	Heart Rate (beats/min)												
	50	60	70	80	90	100	110	120	130	140	150	160	170
Female patients													
3				150	153	157	161	165	169	172	176	180	183
4			141	145	149	152	156	159	163	168	171	175	179
6		130	134	137	142	146	149	153	156	160	165	168	172
8		125	129	133	136	141	144	148	152	155	159	163	167
10	118	122	125	129	133	136	141	144	148	152	155	159	163
12	115	119	122	126	130	133	137	141	145	149	152	156	160
14	112	116	120	123	127	131	134	138	143	146	150	153	157
16	109	114	118	121	125	128	132	136	140	144	148	151	
18	107	111	116	119	123	127	130	134	137	142	146	149	
20	106	109	114	118	121	125	128	132	136	140	144	148	
25	102	106	109	114	118	121	125	128	132	136	140		
30	99	103	106	110	115	118	122	125	129	133	136		
35	97	100	104	107	111	116	119	123	127	130			
50	94	98	102	105	109	112	117	121	124	128			

From LaFarge CG, Miettinen, OS: Cardiovasc Res 4:23, 1970.

INDEX

General guidelines for using this index: Essentially every discussion of a defect or disorder includes a discussion of relevant findings by CXR, ECG, and echocardiography; these are not indexed per individual application. Less common applications like Doppler echo, color flow mapping, and angiocardiography *are* indexed by individual application. Symptoms are not indexed unless a substantive discussion is included or the symptom is unique to the defect or disorder. Consult the drug dosage chart on pp. 307-337 for information on the generic name, brand names, and class type of any given drug; then check under all three for possible references to the drug in the index.

A

Abbokinase, dosage/toxicity, 335

Aberrant right subclavian cavity, 157*f*

Accelerated nodal rhythm, 206-207

Accessory reciprocating AV tachycardia, 202

ACE inhibitors, 250
  for hypertension: dosages, 274*t*
  for myocarditis, 172
  postoperative, 304

Acidosis, 298

Acquired complete heart block, 215

Acquired heart disease, 159-195
  acute rheumatic fever, 179-186
  cardiac tumors, 193-195

cardiovascular infections, 166-175

and congestive heart failure, 243, 244*t*

Kawasaki disease, 175-179

primary myocardial disease, 159-166

valvular heart disease, 186-193

Acute rheumatic fever (*see* Rheumatic fever, acute)

Adalat, dosage/toxicity, 325

Adenocard, dosage/toxicity, 308

Adenosine
  dosage/toxicity, 308
  postoperative, 297
  for supraventricular tachycardia, 240
  for SVC, 203-204

Adrenaline, dosage/toxicity, 317

β-Adrenergic blockers
  for dilated cardiomyopathy, 163
  for hypertension, 273, 274*t*
  for hypertrophic cardiomyopathy, 161